Cell

Monica Grenfell

Cellulite Buster

The 30 Day Diet Plan

PAN BOOKS

First published 2002 by Pan Books
an imprint of Pan Macmillan Ltd
Pan Macmillan, 20 New Wharf Road, London N1 9RR
Basingstoke and Oxford
Associated companies throughout the world
www.panmacmillan.com

ISBN 0 330 49169 5

1 3 5 7 9 8 6 4 2

A CIP catalogue record for this book is available from
the British Library.

Typeset by Intype London Ltd
Printed and bound in Great Britain by
Mackays of Chatham plc, Chatham, Kent

Contents

Introduction

Having cellulite is like wearing your old, grey bra the night you meet Mr Wonderful. It's like breaking your leg during an exercise class and having the paramedics slowly take off your sweaty, smelly leggings and trainers to reveal hairy white legs. On the curl-up-and-die scale it's smashed the glass. Your cover's blown. Cellulite only needs to be seen once for the gossipmongers to get hold of it, then the whole world knows about it and you're shopping for sarongs and desperate for a chance to put the record straight. 'It was a trick of the light!' you cry. Sorry, but we've heard that one before.

Actually, cellulite isn't funny. It's even less funny than legs you're always trying to cover up or a bottom with a mind of its own. It rules your life. While your man's saying, 'Why don't we get up and dance?' you're thinking, 'What made me put on these trousers?' We've all got some body part that fixates us with its awfulness.

I get around 250 letters and e-mails every week, and it appears that for the majority of women thighs are an even bigger obsession than stomachs. Can you believe it? Presumably you can, which is why you've bought this book. People give in to flabby stomachs because they can hide them under long sweaters and baggy tops, but they won't put up with bad legs. Maybe it's because we're so in love with wearing trousers and chafing thighs hurt. Women didn't worry about their thighs half as much years ago when we all wore skirts, and jeans were strictly for gardening. But whatever the reason, you hate your legs and to cap it all you've just discovered they've got cellulite!

When I told people that I was writing this book, they all said, 'But nothing can be done about cellulite, surely? Aren't you just stuck with it?' No you're not. If there's one thing I know, it's that you're never stuck with anything if you don't want to be. The only thing you can't change is your height. Your body is yours, and how it looks is down to you. You can bounce back from a serious illness, regrow a broken nail or restore your split, dry hair back to its former glory. So why not get rid of the cellulite? It takes determination and a good plan, and that's what is in this book. It also takes perseverance. But there's one thing I promise you: it's worth it!

This book is also about getting lovely slim legs and a nice rounded bottom to top it all off. It's possible. Believe me, however far down the road of neglect you've gone, you only have to turn round and face the other way. This year, cellulite, flabby muscles and excess weight are going to be things of the past.

Why are we so worried about our thighs and bottom, parts of the body that spend 90 per cent of the time covered up? For the same reason that we get in a stew about our wedding day. Just because something is once in a lifetime isn't a reason not to bother, and just because a part of us seldom sees the light of day doesn't mean we don't know it's there. And anyway, it's not always covered up. However good your relationships with your loved ones at home, it's not nice to know they're studying your wobbly bits and possibly – just possibly – saying to themselves, '*She's* let herself go a bit.' It doesn't bear thinking about. It's better to strip off and reveal the ace up your sleeve than the joker in the pack. ('My God, did you *see* her on holiday – her body's *amazing!*' has a better ring to it than, 'Did you see her on holiday – she stripped down to her bikini and looked disgusting!' That last observation is usually reserved for women who look enviably immaculate in the office without a hair out of place, who then kick off their shoes to reveal gnarled yellow toenails.)

People love saying that diets don't work, but what alternative is there? They complain about the diet industry but can't come up with anything better which gives no hope to people whose lives are blighted by their weight. Women are encouraged to love themselves whatever size they are – usually by other women who are already slim – but why should you love yourself two stone heavier than you normally are, especially if you've just spent the last twenty years as slim as a rake? It seems to me that right now, a diet is the best we can do.

Diet isn't some magic pill. There isn't a list of food you can just give to someone, and they automatically lose weight. A diet is a whole way of life. In the book I start by looking at how you eat, when you eat and the spacing of your meals. Food is food after all, and there's only so much exercise you can do with two arms and two legs. What's new about my cellulite solution is that I've gone for something that promises both an instant improvement and a long-term plan for the rest of your life. Changing habits is the key to long-term management of cellulite, and I guarantee that once you get rid of it on this plan and get into the long-term changes you've made, you'll never see that cellulite again – ever. This method works – the only other factor is your resolve to keep it up.

My testers loved the Cellulite Buster Diet. At first they thought it went against all the advice they had ever read, which was to eat little and often, to 'graze' and carry healthy snacks in case they got hungry. I had them eating just two main meals a day. They couldn't believe it. Surely they would be hungry? How could they lose weight on large evening meals with cheese to follow? I explained that the fact that they *could* look forward to a substantial evening meal and indeed had to eat it, meant they would eat less during the day. Without that mental get-out clause and the endless negotiating and bargaining with their consciences about what they would give up in order to justify another roast potato, they felt the stressful decisions had been taken away from them. It's amazing how this eliminates obsession and makes waiting for a meal much easier. They began to lose weight, detoxify their bodies and get a much healthier mental attitude to food.

My diet has three great bonuses: it is simple, it works with your body rhythms and it is extremely healthy. You might expect diets to be healthy, but in fact few are. With daily lists of treats that you are supposed to be able to get away with, like crisps or bars of chocolate, or low-calorie, low-fat desserts and cereal bars, most diets are worse for you than what you were eating before! You lose weight on them because there's less food or because the meals are exceptionally low in calories, but they're not nutritious. This diet sets you on the road to total physical improvement because it treats your body well. You'll have better moods and more energy, smoother skin and fat loss. You will begin to love this method of dieting, you will find it easy to stick to and this investment in yourself will pay enormous dividends.

This diet is a complete detoxification programme and I've gone back to basics. No fancy juices or shakes or intricate recipes. No self-indulgent spending on even more food in your quest to actually eat less. While you must treat your body with respect, that doesn't mean obsessive reverence. Nobody needs masses of food and indeed, it is only since food became so available regardless of season that weight problems have got so out of hand. I'm not for one minute saying that you have been greedy, but in a sense I think we have *all* been greedy: we are no longer conscious of how precious food is, and we eat so easily without thinking. The result is cellulite, fat deposits and aches and pains; we can't get up in the morning, have constipation, bad skin, bad breath – the list goes on. If you follow my advice you will be able to restore order to a body that is in chaos.

I want to thank the hundreds of volunteers who tried out the Cellulite Buster Diet. They helped me design the diet: the food you eat is only a part of the story. Meals have to fit in with different schedules – long hours or early starts. Taking food to work in containers or fitting meals in round an elderly relative, managing professional entertaining or coping in a flat with limited cooking facilities – this is where a diet succeeds or fails. I am glad to say it succeeded on all counts because my testers told me what they wanted. They all lost weight, firmed up, banished their cellulite, and were thrilled.

I would like to thank my husband Michael and my sons Michael and James for their total support, my editor Charlie Mounter for being a relentless ray of sunshine and of course the wonderful Gordon Wise for being himself.

Getting started

What is cellulite anyway?

Don't get too wrapped up in this one. I'm not sure that anybody really cares what it is and certainly it doesn't make having it any more bearable. Men are said not to care if we have it and babies are apparently all born with dimpled bottoms. Do men have cellulite? I haven't looked. I would rather concentrate on your cellulite and what we are going to do about it!

There are so many theories about cellulite, and none of them have been proven. I asked many experts what cellulite is, notably physiotherapists and osteopaths who see hundreds of pairs of legs every year in their clinics, as they massage and manipulate and apply electrodes and I don't know what to various injuries. They feel the cellulite under their fingers. What is it? It's fat, it's fluid-filled sacs, it's ropey muscle and it's slack skin. The slack skin happens anyway, as we get older, and to a small degree the creams and scrubs and potions we all love to dismiss actually do have a slight cosmetic effect on smoothing the surface of the skin – the problem is that the effect doesn't last very long. So what about the fat?

The fat isn't special. It is normal body fat but it has a different appearance because it lies very close to the skin's surface. It collects in pockets and then, as we sit on it, it gets squashed. The average person exerts a mind-boggling 35 kilos of pressure on it for many hours as they sit working or resting. Spare calories are converted into fat stores and down they go – right to the nether regions where they won't be disturbed. Then there's the ropey muscle element. Whether you used to be fit or have never been fit, underused muscles can look thick, knobbly or knotted, like a piece of overstretched, perished elastic. The combination of fat beneath the skin's surface, flabby, underused muscles and slack skin all add up to cellulite!

Fluid-filled, retentive sacs are the source of a lot of controversy in medical and dietary circles. Women do retain a lot of fluid in the thigh and buttock region, but excess, retained fluid can be easily disposed of with a high-fibre, high-water diet. Hormones are the root cause of this strictly female experience, and all menstruating women retain fluid from mid cycle onwards. But don't worry, in my last book *The Beat Your Body Chaos Diet* I discussed hormones from start to finish, so if you need to know anything about the worst times for hormonal activity and the way to combat their effects, rush out and buy this book straight away for all the explanations. Fluid retention is also a direct result of a poor diet and poor gastric emptying or constipation. Chemical overload is another reason. Even if you think you have a healthy diet from low-fat, low-calorie special ready-meal ranges that promise 'no additives!' I would be very wary of those misleading claims. One look at pages 51–2 will tell you what's hidden in supposedly healthy chicken breast fillets, and the minute you've got emulsifiers or gelling agents in food, you've got chemicals. My diet bans all these sorts of meals. As long as you can make the commitment to real food, plenty of fibre and plenty of potassium which helps rid you of excess fluid, you're giving your body its best-ever chance of busting that cellulite for good.

The Cellulite Buster is your emergency rescue plan. With a brilliant fat-burning, calorie-restricted diet which will force those extra fat stores into action, and with a lot of exercise, you'll have truly impressive results. Power walking, swimming or cycling are essential. You don't have to do all of them, but power walking is best if you can manage only one activity. It'll blast that cellulite and get those ropey muscles going again. You're on your way!

Help! I've let myself go!

Nobody ever just woke up fat. Nobody had smooth legs one day and cellulite the next. Your body is a growing, changing thing and cellulite happened while you were busy doing something else. While you were happily thinking you were OK, and everyone was amazed and jealous at how lucky you were to smoke and eat fast food and look so fabulous, your cellulite was in the post. Your thighs got flabby when you were having that great romance, moving house or cramming for your exams. So who's perfect? I understand that bodies are a lot of hard work and if it's not one thing it's another. But only you can deal with it. You need to put failure behind you, not get bogged down with what used to be. Concentrate on the solution.

Women who let themselves go say they haven't time to stay looking good. But it's more likely that they aren't trying as hard as they should. Often their attempts at weight loss and exercise are half-hearted. They go through manic phases of eating kilos of fruit and wearing out the treadmill, then they don't do anything for weeks on end. Their age or their personal circumstances affect their resolve. They think that they can't expect to have cellulite-free legs after having two children. They're not surprised that nothing happens because they didn't expect much in the first place and it reinforces their beliefs. They were right to think that they couldn't look good, so this whole process becomes a self-fulfilling prophecy. They are quick to blame their age when their thighs are spreading, saying that they aren't teenagers any more, or that nobody over thirty-five has the legs they used to have. But that's rubbish. They say that metabolism 'automatically' slows down into the thirties and forties, and a person's weight is expected to rise, but that's rubbish too. It is fashionable for diet writers to tell of their amazing battles with weight problems, and how their success story was their inspiration to write a book, but I'm sorry to report that I haven't such a sad story to draw upon.

I'm not even half a kilo heavier now than I was in 1975. Apart from pregnancy, the needle hasn't slipped one way or the other. While you might dismiss this as my being lucky or naturally slim, I'm afraid it's neither. I haven't gained weight because I decided I wasn't going to. I ate this diet. I ate twice a day just as I'm going to recommend you do, and I was careful. It's not some miracle or fantastic luck. Like everyone over the age of forty-five I expected a few pounds to creep on sometime or another and they haven't. Don't ever think you can't expect much because you can. I reckoned that if it worked for me, it could work for anyone.

So decide that you're going to be slim, ignore the doom-mongers and expect to look good. Busy-busy lives are a fact of life, and while there's a clear difference between the single girl living alone in a low-maintenance flat and the working mother of five, the trick is to organize yourself along labour-saving lines. It is hard to admit that you can't find time for yourself, especially if you consider yourself efficient. This is how I've made it easy:

— The diet has limited choice – with a basis of fruits, vegetables, nuts, grains and seeds, your shopping list will be smaller and decision-making a thing of the past.
— The diet is in two separate phases – with an optional fast-track week if you're really struggling with motivation.
— Each main meal has savoury options, including a cheese course.
— All your food preparation can be done in less than an hour, once a week. Then it's just a case of dishing it out.
— No time needed for travelling to the gym, parking and changing. Most exercise is activity-based or done at home.
— No time-wasting cellulite cures. This beauty plan is simple, and effective.

You'll lose weight

Not everyone who has cellulite also needs to lose weight, but if you are more than 6 kilos over your ideal weight, expect to shed between 4.5 to 6 kilos over the initial thirty days of the diet. To be sure that the weight comes off your legs and bottom, don't neglect your top half but concentrate instead on diverting the energy from your meals to the musclestructure of your chest, back and arms, thus making sure you lose inches below the waist. Losing weight will make you lighter – exercise will make your new figure noticeable.

Changing for the better – old habits die hard

How often have you said that diets don't work? How easy it is to say it! But what does that mean? That you did a diet and didn't lose an ounce? You lost a bit of weight and then lost no more? Lost a lot and put it all back on again?

It seems to me that the people who dismiss diets as 'not working' are under the same illusions as people who get angry about cosmetic surgery. They think that weight loss will change their lives. Losing weight will make you lighter, but it won't necessarily make you more attractive. Losing your cellulite won't make you a better person; it won't turn back time or get you that job you wanted, although it will make you look much, much better, and with luck, top up your confidence and put the smile back on your face. Life is about a bit more than where the needle stops on the scales, and when life doesn't magically come up with the goods the minute you reach your goal weight, many people go back to the chocolate cake and the weight problem. 'Diets are rubbish,' they scoff.

People might also say a diet doesn't work when they finish it and go back to old eating habits. The weight comes back because they have gone back to being the person they were before. So two *better* goals are slimming and habit changes. Slimming will help you look better, younger, fitter and firmer. Your diet will help you to slim down a dress size and lose unsightly fat in your hip and bottom areas, while if you change your habits and exercise this will tone, lengthen and refine your muscle structure. New presentation skills will help you look glossier and more confident as well as showing yourself in the best light. So while it remains the first few steps on the ladder to success and is certainly not a cure-all for your problems, this mental picture of a better 'you' emerging should help to keep you going. You won't want to blow it all for the sake of five minutes with a piece of cake.

This book is my plan for the perfect lower half. I have used it with countless clients over the years, and they all report that they are still cellulite-free and have smaller appetites. And this is the true test of success: it is one thing to lose the weight and get into a size ten: it's quite another to keep it up. You don't want to spend your life feeling that you're 'on a diet', but you can be on a diet and not know it. Beauty is an entire effect, so getting a diet that is your personal signature is like having a certain dress- or hairstyle. In the same way that you might say 'I'm a blonde' or 'I'm happier in jeans', you should add 'I don't eat between meals' or 'I never touch sweet things'.

If you find this hard, think of it as playing a role. At some stage in your life, you realize you're identified with outdated circumstances. You're stuck with your past. It's like you once used to buy a certain brand of cosmetics and used your store reward card when paying, not knowing that they use this to compile information on your buying habits. Then you change. You stop wearing make-up, you go upmarket, downmarket, get married, who knows what? Have a facelift. You don't want that stuff you used to buy any more. But month after month their promotional junk literature comes banging through the post. You're on their system, in their clutches. 'That was then!' you want to shout. 'I hate cosmetics now. I'm not that person any longer.' Well, sorry, but they've got you down as a cosmetics person.

This is what happens with diets, and especially with the people who know you well. It's what happens with yourself. If you've lost weight before and gained it again, maybe you are associating yourself with someone you used to be. Maybe you are like the store computer system, and you've labelled yourself not the slim type. 'I know I can never be a size twelve,' someone will say to me, 'but I'd be happy to settle for a fourteen or small sixteen.' Why? Why can't someone be a size twelve, or more to the point, what has happened in someone's life to persuade her that she can never be so slim? I'll tell you what happened: other people got hold of her and told her so, or she lost weight and didn't look as good as she'd hoped. The frocks still didn't fit. Her stomach still looked huge. She still had cellulite and that pouchy look in her lower abdomen. Or maybe the regimes she chose were wrong for her or she hadn't the willpower. The list goes on but it illustrates my point, I think, that getting lighter and seeing each lost pound as a fabulous achievement is somehow missing the point. If you still keep the mind of the old you, things will go back to where they were before. Your old mind thought you were hopeless at dieting. The old you needed snacks and worried a week ahead of a long car journey about what food you'd take or where the service stations were located. The old you bought food you thought you *might* need, not food you needed. When you went shopping you had a mental checklist of things for the storecupboard, like crisps, cereal bars and cakes. They're habits. And if you don't change these habits at the same time that you change your body, you'll find the same old problems coming back time and again.

Other people don't help. 'Oh, she's got a massive appetite,' I once heard a mother say of her thirty-four-year-old daughter, who had lost 36 kilos in eighteen months. 'She needs her food. She's got a terribly sweet tooth, so I make her her favourite coffee and walnut cake anyway, every weekend. She always has a slice or two.' Er, no. She used to have a massive appetite. That's what got her into that mess. She's eating two slices of your cake because she daren't do anything else. Why don't you do something for her and recognize that she's changed?

My usual glib answer is simply to get a new set of friends and start with a clean sheet, but realistically you can't just shunt everyone out of your life and not see them again. But getting a new diet for yourself and *believing* in it is a challenge. It's especially a challenge if you actually love your weekly fish and chips, curry or nightly half bottle of wine, don't want to give them up, but know that you have to. How can you convince yourself and others that you really are happier with half an avocado pear?

There's no getting away from the fact that things must change. I wish that I could be one of these diet writers who gives you daily treats. I wish I could find weakness and lapses and bingeing amusing. I wish I could give you lists of food that you can have 'unlimited' amounts of. I'd love to be able to say, 'Carry around some healthy snacks in case you get peckish.' But I can't do any of these things, simply because I don't believe in them. I want you to get rid of cellulite, firm up and lose weight, and I know you can't do that successfully unless you go for it with some seriousness.

Treating your body from the inside out

We've all bought ourselves treats. A squashy cream cake, a bag of pretzels or a Mars bar. But to your body it's not a treat at all. This invasion of sugar, sludge and chemicals is a massive stress on your body. A proper treat, something for which your body would be grateful if only it could tell you so, would be a bowl of fruit salad, a banana or a stick of celery. These things make your body clean and healthy because they are high in fibre and fibre cleanses your gut. It's all very well to spend time and money on creams and lotions and days of pampering at health spas, but they're papering over the cracks. The idea with the Cellulite Buster Diet is that the cracks don't appear in the first place. Eating properly and well is a necessity. When you sit down to eat your plate of salad and chicken I want you to think about what it's doing for you: helping your muscles, skin and hair to grow better; helping to thoroughly cleanse your system. I think that if you can learn to concentrate on the goodness of your meals, and celebrate this, you will come a long way to loving this way of eating for ever.

Try to spend whatever money you can afford on the best food. It won't cost more in the long run because once you get rid of crisps and biscuits, the savings will be fantastic. Some critics think this encourages obsession. But it isn't obsessive to want better hair, to get rid of dandruff and split ends or stop your nails flaking. Hairdressing shops and beauty salons line every high street in the country, but nobody thinks it odd or obsessive to wage war on your split ends. It isn't weird to want to make the most of your body, so go for it. Don't let anybody put you off.

Although this is a thirty-day diet, there's only so much I can get into one book. Ideally, I'd like to write something to keep you going for the next thirty years, but this method at least sets you on your way and gives you a plan for the future. You might be pleased with the results as they stand, or you might want to go further. You might *need* to go further. There's an obvious difference between the person who's just discovered her once-lovely legs are looking a bit iffy, and the person who is trying to undo years of neglect. Don't worry, because I've explained how to carry on the diet in the future, so you can plan as many months ahead as you like and not worry that being on a diet will get in the way of Christmas or holidays. It's a complete way of living. After all, to listen to the propaganda you'd think that everyone gained weight at Christmas and on holiday and everyone went on a diet in January and May. Not so. If you're one of the people who dreams of being the same weight all the time, with no separate sets of 'fat' and 'thin' clothes and no automatic five-kilo weight gain at Christmas, the Cellulite Buster Diet will work for you. Your weight always goes back to your natural body weight, if you've had an established, steady regime beforehand. This is why my diet is a complete way of living, because it will flatten out those ups and downs in your life. You won't have to go through this agony of cellulite and weight gain and loss ever again.

Thirty days? Isn't that just a quick fix?

No, it's a quick start. Like taking antibiotics for a chest infection you'll get better in a week, but if you took nothing you'd still get better – except it would take longer. You'd lose 12 kilos in twelve months if you walked a bit more and cut out the odd piece of cake, but you can speed this up by doubling the walking effort and adding a few gym sessions and eating 500 calories fewer per day. Those two stone would be gone in three months. The end result would be the same but you would have doubled your efforts, and this is what the thirty days is about. It's a short cut, it will cheer you up and give you the motivation to keep going and it's very,

very effective. But what you have to do is keep it up for the future, and there's no short cut to that.

Thirty days on a sustained, focused plan will see your lower half shaping up and melting away into a smaller, firmer, smoother bottom and thighs. If your holiday is next month you can go all-out for the fast-track option, but if your next really big event is six months away, you can get into it quickly in thirty days, then settle into the coasting programme and lose weight the gradual way. It doesn't matter and it doesn't make the process any easier, but it *does* give you that psychological boost when you have such a great result in just a month.

OK, most body processes take the same length of time, which is why you can't make your hair or nails grow any faster. But you can do an awful lot to make them *look* longer. Cuticle care, volumizing mousses for your hair – even wearing different clothes or putting on fake tan. You can't change nature but you *can* influence it. Trust me, thirty days is quite enough time to blast that cellulite and get thinner thighs and a gorgeous bottom!

Don't lose the big picture

Don't get caught up in the downside of a diet. The small things you're giving up (choc ices, quick microwaved meals) are far outweighed by the advantages. Concentrate on those. Crossing a pair of slender legs that don't rub together. Walking away from people in a pair of jeans and not feeling fifty pairs of eyes burning into your backside. The sheer confidence of wearing a swimming costume. Enjoying an elegant, modest, nutritious meal feels better than fish and chips. Honestly. Tell me when someone has said no to chips, eaten salad instead and woken up next day kicking herself. It just doesn't happen.

The first step to achieving anything is determination that you're going to get it. No settling for half measures. No 'I can't expect much at my age' or 'I'll be pleased to just look better'. Women who dread big thighs don't get them. It isn't about being obsessed or spending half the day exercising or giving up chocolate for ever. Looking good doesn't have to be a fight, it doesn't have to be about denial and it isn't about hard work and expense. It's about setting your thoughts on looking after yourself and seeing this as a forward move. Every day you will be getting

– and looking – better, not worse. You *are* going to get the most beautiful lower half you've ever wanted, lose weight and banish cellulite, and you mustn't settle for any less.

How the plan works

There are three elements to this programme: diet, exercise and presentation. The diet has three phases, first to get you started slowly, next to achieve maximum weight loss and discipline and, finally, a plan for the future.

Just for the record

This first step is important. Take any sort of photo of your rear view (be it Polaroid or normal snap), and stick it on the page opposite.

You need to record how you look now, otherwise you won't know how much you have improved once you've been on the diet. You're not going to look at your backside AT ALL for the next thirty days, not in a full-length mirror, not a glance behind you, nothing. You'll want to check and see if anything earth-shattering is happening, but you mustn't. Wait thirty days and then compare the results with your photo.

Here are the basic rules for a flawless shot:

— Wear a G-string or nothing at all.
— Don't use flash – this has the handy habit of smoothing out all lumps and bumps and being incredibly flattering, which is not what we're after just now! Stand in normal, clear light, preferably daylight by a window. Don't stand in sunlight either – this also smoothes out any lumps!
— Don't lean forward or bend over. Stand completely straight, with your weight equally on both feet.
— Have your feet together or nearly together – but not far apart.
— Take three shots of the same pose – in case one doesn't come out.

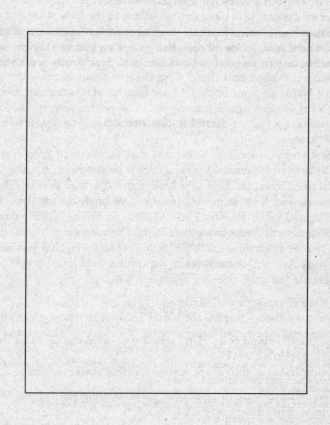

Weighing and measuring

In my book *Fabulous in a Fortnight* I suggested that readers measure themselves in many places, including round their wrists and the tops of their arms, and I left a blank page for these measurements to be recorded. The book came out first in 1995 and I have lost count of the number of women who have written to me in the past year to say that they either had a baby, went to work abroad, had a serious illness or whatever, and had no idea if they had gained weight or changed shape, or whether they really used to be as slim as they remembered, then they had found my book and there were their measurements and weekly weights! 'Without your book I'd have had no idea what my measurements were six years ago,' someone wrote to me the other week. So now here you have a page to record for all time what your figure was *really* like this year:

Date	Waist	Top of thigh	R	L
Weight	Navel	Mid-thigh	R	L
Height	Pubic bone	Above knee	R	L
	Full part of hips			

To recap

— Put failure behind you – don't spend time thinking about all the diets that didn't work.
— Concentrate on your shape and size, rather than every kilo gained or lost.
— You weren't born with cellulite – so you can get rid of it.
— Thirty days is a quick start.
— Decide on success.
— Losing the big picture – don't get sidetracked or seduced out of your motivation.

The
Cellulite Buster
Diet

The rules

Food

— All food must be fresh.
— VEGETABLES must be the highest-fibre food you have. Choose vegetables with a shell or skin, like beans and peas. However, all vegetables are good.
— ONE or TWO portions of chicken, fish or eggs should be eaten every day.
— BREAD should only be eaten for breakfast.
— POTATOES should only be eaten for dinner.
— ASPARAGUS and CELERY should be eaten every day as a salad.
— ALL desserts should be fruit in some form or another.
— Choose fruit with a STONE, or BERRIES.
— NO white bread, white rice or pasta.

Eating

— TWO main meals a day.
— ONE lighter meal a day.
— Only FOUR items on the plate – one high protein, three vegetable.
— Two SAVOURY courses are an option.

Exercise

— Thirty minutes should be spent on a specific exercise, every day.
— In addition, you should have a THIRTY-MINUTE (minimum) walk every day.

The Diet

I have divided the thirty-day main diet into two phases to help you get the best from your biological rhythms. It works with them, providing energy when you need it, re-stocking fuel and making sure your blood-sugar levels are high enough to give you a good night's sleep. After all, it's not much good having legs to die for if you're so whacked you're in bed before the party starts!

Phase One – the first thirty days

Most people go into overdrive when they start a new diet. Long shopping lists, new trainers and a yoga mat by the door. There's a 'last supper' where everything and anything is consumed and drunk in vast quantities. Then D-day dawns and it's nothing to eat and a halo round the head as the weight drops off. Boy, does it feel good.

Unfortunately that's about as good as it gets. Energy doesn't last, the fabulous weight loss of the first week slows to nothing and by week three you're wondering why you should go to all the bother if your weight won't budge.

Well, you always did say that diets don't work.

However saintly you feel about being so good, this sort of dieting is just a monumental shock for your body and hard to keep up. You are going too fast, too soon.

This Cellulite Buster Diet won't put a stress on your body. During the first thirty days your cellulite will get a hammering from exercise and salt scrubs and the diet is the support system. It will nourish your new cells, help drain away excess fluids and detoxify your system of all those chemicals, and it will challenge your body to use its fat stores. To do this, you need nutritious, plain food and lots of water.

I've given you menu ideas with a lot of variety, but if you're keen to get off with a real bang and don't mind a simple diet, do make up your own menus from the recommended foods in the section So What Am I Going to Eat?

Remember that the idea is to force your body to use those stores of fat and cellulite you hate so much, and every time you feel hungry, your body is going to turn to your excess weight for fuel. I know this is the hardest bit and, mindful that this could be a challenge for you, I've given you a few ideas about dealing with difficulties in the section Cravings, Tricky Situations and Setbacks (see page 96). Remember, half the problem is discarding old habits, but new ones are adopted amazingly quickly. A smoker doesn't keep craving cigarettes with the same intensity for years on end!

However, I don't want to focus on an imagined downside. You might not have cravings and you won't feel this is torture. If a diet does have you feeling you can't cope, it's a bad diet. The whole point of the Cellulite Buster Diet is that it works with your body rhythms and won't have you helpless with hunger. So please don't get it into your head that this is going to be some kind of torture. Getting a fabulous body is anything *but* torture.

Phase Two – coasting

This happens after thirty days on the Cellulite Buster plan. Phase Two is called coasting because this is what you'll be doing. You'll have got a grip on your eating habits, learned a little better how to manage your shopping and cooking and most important of all – you'll have a total grip on willpower. That's the important bit! Phase Two allows you to have those extra calories, as long as you're still exercising. If you feel your weight loss sliding or even going up a bit, don't worry – you can go straight back to Phase One.

Coasting will be effortless. Coasting means observing the rules you have already learned and adapting them so you can go out and enjoy yourself with a drink or two, a four-course meal if necessary or a fattening tea at your sister-in-law's without that sinking guilt or panic the next morning. In other words you won't need willpower.

Your day off

You'll also be able to have a weekly 'splurge' day (which doesn't mean binge!). It allows good things you might be missing, like red meat or pasta, but it's not an excuse to eat junk! That phase of your life will now be over. You'll trust yourself and know that chemicals and manufactured food are evil for your body. You'll be so proud of yourself when you get into the coasting stage, you won't want to ruin all your hard work. In other words, eating beautifully will be second nature!

Detoxing

Your body doesn't need special detox diets. It does the job admirably by itself, but sometimes we don't help the process by eating a lot of sludge or eating nothing at all. Sweating, urinating and fat loss are all ways to get rid of waste. Exercise, fluids and a calorie-restricted diet are the solution to an overloaded, over-burdened body. You can be carrying up to 5 kilos of non-fat waste inside you, caused by a build-up of fluids and delayed gastric emptying. I know it's not an elegant topic of conversation, but it's one we all have to face. I talk about this later in the section on fibre, but you'll be amazed at how brilliant you'll start to feel when your natural detox systems get working properly again with this diet.

Exercise

Exercise – not a cure for eating

The modern love–hate relationship with exercise has become a stressful trade-off and bargaining process. 'If I spend an hour in the gym, I can eat chips/have two glasses of wine today,' has become the alternative to just saying no. Diets *do* work, but only if you do them. Trust me, the only way to get slim, stay slim and stop being anxious, despairing and depressed about your weight is to eat less and eat differently. Bargaining with that little voice in your head about whether you can have a cereal bar if you go for a walk afterwards, does more harm than good.

I don't bother with gym-based exercise in this book, but if you love it, keep going. Gyms can be fantastic places if you find them motivational and social, but exercise isn't a cure for eating. Don't spend time staring granite-faced at a gym wall. Activity is central to the war against cellulite and flabby thighs, but not with gadgets and meters and TV screens to stave off boredom as you tramp miles on a treadmill in a depressing row with twenty others. I can't think of anything worse than paying to go for a walk indoors. Get moving, get supple and get strong. Be active!

Exercise is more than a calorie-burning process. It tones your muscles and speeds up your circulation. The pounding heart, heavy breathing and extra sweating that result from exercise all promote the most wonderful detoxification and help with the removal of carbon dioxide and excess fluids. A mix of all types of exercise is vital in the quest for a cellulite-free body and gorgeous toned legs and buttocks.

Muscles move all the time, but usually we use only a fraction of their range. Exercise that tones and stretches your muscles gets deep to the root of good physical function. You'll be putting your thigh and buttock muscles through their paces with the exercises I suggest, and this will get everything moving again to blast those fat deposits right out of your body.

Fat is no more than a waste product. You might call it storage fat for emergency energy, but 20 kilos of excess fat is an emergency in itself. If you are gradually laying down more and more fat, it means your balance of energy has gone a bit lopsided. Don't beat yourself up about this but be aware of that gradual slide away from activity and into the odd snack. There's a lot of hype around about larger dress sizes being 'real' and while I don't think there's anything to be ashamed about, it seems to have given people the green light to be very overweight and see it as OK. It's true that you can look as sexy and appealing as anyone else, and there's no doubt that many men prefer bigger women, but it never has been and never will be healthy to have a lot of body fat. To be healthy, you must be lean.

These are the exercises you will be doing:

— fast walking
— stair running or stepping
— leg exercises lying on the floor or standing
— swimming (optional)
— cycling (optional)
— aerobics (optional)
— stretching

Presentation

If you're following this diet so you can strip off on the beach or clinch the deal with a potential new man, you'll be extra-sensitive about your nether regions. You can't always count on good or sympathetic lighting if the mood suddenly strikes, and although they say that men don't mind about lumps and bumps, we do. If you feel self-conscious, the deal's off. Some cellulite solutions work, others aren't worth wasting your money on. I'll be giving you a daily plan to help improve how you present yourself which you must stick with for best results, and I'll also be saving you a lot of time and hassle by recommending a good salt-scrub treatment for your thighs which you make up yourself.

This regime is based on my personal experience, and the experience of friends and product testers who have helped me. Basically, very few products are worthwhile, but a daily regime will make all the difference between looking OK and looking amazing. We can't all look like glamorous Hollywood stars, but I think you owe it to yourself to make the most of what you've got. Looking like you've made an effort does more for you than wearing the entire Paris spring collection. Looking happy and proud of yourself says more than a carrier bag full of Chanel cosmetics. A facelift's not much good on a miserable face. Striding out with good, toned, waxed and glossy legs will do more for your reputation than a pair of thin, cellulite-free pins with a pair of grubby feet at the end of them. Just make sure to treat your legs and bottom like gold dust, and they will pay you back richly in terms of compliments and self-assurance.

How to eat – the secret of the Cellulite Buster Diet

Success isn't just about the food you eat. The real secret is in the way you eat, how you think of your meals, how they are spaced, the portion size, how long it takes you to eat and, of course, your attitude as a whole. Bargaining with yourself to justify that chocolate bar isn't the way forward. Food is your fuel for life and limb, not some sort of calorie bank balance that you have to pay back with a long run round the block. If you eat properly, eat simply and value your meals, you won't ever have to worry about your weight again, I promise.

Being able to control your appetite isn't just a matter of being preoccupied or off your food so that you don't want to eat; a balanced, steady diet with no missed meals and enough carbohydrate and protein will help your brain chemicals adjust to accepting a controlled way of eating and make you less inclined to binge or feel hungry. A sugary, high-starch diet can lead to highs and lows in blood sugar, and crash dieting or long periods without food can lead to muddled thinking, gnawing hunger and feverish eating. The best thing about this diet is that it calms your mind and your appetite, and the people who tested it for me were amazed that their lust for food simply vanished after two or three days.

People who worry about getting fat usually start by missing meals. They skip breakfast, with the promise to themselves that they will eat when they get to the office or when they get back from dropping the children off at school. Then after a morning spent sustained by diet colas and strong coffee, lunch is also relegated to an insubstantial snack: an apple and a cereal bar, a banana or a low-fat yoghurt. When asked if she is going to lunch, the slimmer will reply that she has a special meal to go to tonight, so she is 'saving' herself for it. Breakfast is missed because of the huge meal she had the night before. This becomes an exercise in bargaining. 'Is it OK if I have a massive meal tonight where I eat three times my normal intake? I promise I'll have no lunch!' (Forgetting of course that her lunch might have had 300 calories, but she intends eating an extra 1,000 calories tonight – the maths never adds up.)

You know that awful feeling when you've simply had too much to eat – the subtle undoing of the trouser button, the loosening of the zip. When you get to this stage, you've overdone it, but more than that, this type of eating is crazy. Your body is designed to cope with large meals, but that comes from the days when we might have had only one major meal every two days and nothing in between. Quite simply, none of us need worry much about where the next meal is coming from, so why the need to cram in so much in one go? If you are going to look good, you should learn to eat more modest portions!

Food eaten 'out of context' is important because it is always the calories you don't remember eating that cause the problems. If only I had a pound for every time someone has written to me, 'I have a bowl of cereal at 6.30 a.m., then I don't eat again until 2.30 p.m. when I have a small salad sandwich. I then can't stop for anything until the evening when I share a meal of maybe fish or chicken with a small jacket potato and vegetables. I hardly ever have chocolate except perhaps once a week, no sickly puddings and if I have chips, just a few. Despite this, I have steadily gained 6 kilos each year, and now weigh 50 kilos.'

Anybody believe her?

You see, it isn't that people are being untruthful. It is like trying to say accurately what you spent last week. You remember the big things you bought but not the odd magazine or the car-parking ticket you got. It's staggering how incidental bits of food add up and that is why incidental eating must be banned.

You must stick rigidly to my methods of cooking and eating, which are outlined on page 55–8. Let's start with what you are going to eat, and why it is important to stick with this diet for weight loss and cellulite-busting success.

Eat two main meals a day

How often have you started a diet only to find your good intentions vanishing by the evening? It's easy to eat less in the daytime when you've got plenty to do, but hard to manage on a tiny plateful at night. Some people say it's due to boredom, I call it nature. In times gone by, when the sun went down in winter it meant going to bed as early as 6 o'clock. There weren't any candles and the fire had to be saved. You could be asleep for fourteen or sixteen hours which meant eating as much as possible for your last meal of the day. On waking, you would have needed another substantial meal. There were no store cupboards to raid, no little snacks of chocolate to nibble on if you got a bit peckish. Every meal counted. I am convinced that we were designed to eat large amounts when the daylight starts to fade, and that we want to eat more in winter for these reasons. With artificial light we can cheat our body clocks, but eating two good meals a day remains my recipe for stable bodyweight.

In case you think that life has moved on and we have overridden our primitive eating patterns, consider how your body works: your appendix and tonsils have no use, but the rest is exactly the same as it would have been several thousand years ago. We haven't evolved with a different digestion. We haven't evolved so we can do without sleep or manage on less water. Every single working bit of our bodies is the same as when we were eating meat and berries, which is why it's hard to cope on mind-boggling amalgamations of food like burgers and pizzas. Wind, bloating, vague aches and pains, inability to wake up in the morning, inability to sleep – ever heard of a bird who can't get up in the morning? Sheep who feel irritable? That's because they live and eat as they've always done.

No more 'grazing'

This brings me on neatly to grazing. Grazing and snacking have become the background to society, but you're not a grazing animal! The argument used by some experts in favour of grazing and against main meals is that main meals send too big a load of carbohydrates, fats and proteins into your body at the same time. I would argue that this only happens when you have eaten the typical Sunday-lunch-type meal, say roast meat, roast potatoes and parsnips, a fat and sugar pudding like fruit crumble and custard, washed down with half a bottle of wine. Even if it's just pasta, ice cream and a couple of bottles of beer, it's the same thing. The load is huge. Fat, sugar and protein on an empty stomach send your system into overdrive. The alternative solution is a system of 'grazing' on five or six small meals a day, usually nibbled fruit, cereal bars or yoghurt. I can't see that this suits us at all.

When you look at the three main types of eating pattern you'll see how we should work with our natural eating rhythms:

Grazing – where you eat food that is available. Grazing animals, like cows and sheep, eat grass, fruits, leaves and seeds – all vegetable matter. They provide so few calories that the animals have to eat non-stop to fuel their energy, but they move very little in the course of a day.

Foraging – you unearth or seek out your food. Birds are foragers and scratch or dig for seeds, worms or insects which are high in proteins and fats and potentially provide many calories. However, the energy needed to fly or walk around to find the food means the energy benefits are almost cancelled out. Feeding is constant and sleeping time is minimal. Birds are always up with the dawn, trying to keep pace with their energy needs for flying.

Hunting – you go looking for your food. Animals that hunt eat once or twice a day and in between times, they rest. The huge calorie benefits from each kill provide energy for half a day, so there is no need to eat in between times. Cats, dogs and birds of prey are hunters, and spend many hours resting, idle or sleeping off their last meal.

Humans are hunters. The food you eat directly fuels your energy needs. People get fat when they eat like hunters but forage and graze as well, on foods with a high fat and sugar content, like biscuits. The energy value of a high-protein meal should last half a day, so a small meal between the two main meals should be of the low-calorie foraging variety, foods like seeds, leaves and fruit, which is why your diet specifies salad for lunch.

On this diet, your main meals will be breakfast and dinner, and they should be eaten between nine and twelve hours apart. You should have a light lunch and plenty to drink in the form of water or milk. On the whole, people give in to, or panic about feeling hungry in a way that is totally out of proportion to the problem. Nobody is ever far from food. It's not as if you've got a ten-mile trek in deep snow before you can get to a meal. If you have excess body fat, you can manage a few hunger pangs. Here are a few rules:

— Don't carry snacks around with you.
— Never miss meals.
— Never go without a meal to try to lose that extra half pound.
— Do build up a nice appetite for your main meals, and try not to spoil them by snacking.
— It is important to eat slow-release carbohydrates, and I have plenty of ideas for meals with foods which release their energy over several hours, rather than giving you an instant boost followed by a downer.

Fuelling and re-stocking – lighting that fire

Burning calories isn't just about the food you eat. It's also about the body you put it in. Your body's like a fire that needs lighting and stoking. If you have a fire that you want to quietly stay in all day, you keep it alight with small amounts of dry fuel. Tip a load of big damp logs onto it and you'll put it out. Dry fuel is like putting cotton wool into a furnace. Think of your body in the same way. In the morning your hormone levels are high, preparing you for the day ahead. Food eaten at this time is burnt quickly, so you can eat a lot more low-sugar carbohydrates at this time. They're needed!

During the day your fire needs to be kept in without being damped down. Do this with a light lunch. Nothing heavy, especially no sugar. Refined sugar is completely banned on this diet, especially sugar combined with fat, in, for example, biscuits, pastry and cakes.

In the evening you need to keep the fire in all night. Forget about not eating carbohydrates after 6 p.m. or whatever. Forget anything you've heard about stodge being laid down as fat. It's rubbish. You have to get through at least twelve hours before you eat again, and your body will be empty of energy. Re-stock your body before 9 p.m. to keep that fire in all night, and you'll wake refreshed. Trust me. If you ever wake in the night feeling edgy and then can't wake in the morning, that's low blood sugar. You've not eaten enough for dinner.

The metabolism question

It is often argued that eating only two or three times a day slows the metabolism. This isn't quite true. Metabolic rate rises slightly whenever food is eaten, but it also rises in response to shivering, smoking or fidgeting. Eating is an activity that requires energy, but you have to remember that one activity cancels out the other. While eating raises your metabolism, at the same time you are ingesting calories, so in one sense you are giving with one hand and taking away with the other. As I have said, animals graze because the food they graze on has so few calories, they have to keep eating to stay ahead of their energy balance. Eating is an energy- or calorie-burning process, but it is not strictly true that it raises your metabolism. This would mean your resting energy-burning rate was raised permanently, and this is not what happens when you eat. The few calories burned in the process of eating are easily cancelled out by the energy of the food itself. Metabolism is permanently raised only by the amount of lean tissue in your body, which is linked to your age. Two main meals a day, with a top-up in between, is the basis for success.

Note to diabetics

Many diabetics ask if this diet is suitable for them. As I have one son who is an insulin-dependent diabetic, I feel I can answer with confidence. He has reduced his insulin units dramatically through control of sugar and starchy foods, and the basis of his present diet is carbohydrates from vegetables, milk and yoghurt and some fruit. He has added one small snack to the meals I have suggested, but has not found the need to eat more frequently. This diet is suitable for diabetics, as long as you have the approval of your doctor or diabetic nurse.

Breakfast

It's an interesting fact that if you had a plate of cereal for your evening meal you'd think you hadn't eaten much. Yet people often tell me that they have a bowl of cornflakes for breakfast every morning, maybe even followed by a piece of fruit, and – lo and behold! – they're hungry again by mid-morning! Is anybody surprised?

Breakfast is a main meal. You probably don't allow the same time for it that you do for dinner, but you should. Those extra minutes in bed aren't needed if you eat properly the night before, and if you can't wake up in the morning and feel woolly-headed, you didn't eat enough the night before. Low blood sugar is a prime cause of restlessness in the early hours and the inability to wake up in the morning. If you eat two good meals a day, you won't suffer this again.

Breakfast is your high-carbohydrate, high-protein first main meal of the day and you must eat within an hour of waking. This is what I recommend:

Bread – eat bread at this meal, but not at any other. You can only have it with a protein addition like an egg or some cheese. You should also have a banana.

Oats – you can have oats in any form, but you need to add nuts, seeds and banana to an oat-based cereal.

Don't try to last out on a quick slice of toast and marmalade. If you're rushing, get up twenty minutes earlier. If you can't get up early because you're always shattered from the night before, go to bed earlier!

Lunch

'Lunch is for wimps' was a popular cry of the swaggering classes in the 1980s and 90s. It sounded clever, and anyway, they never actually went without lunch; they were usually found some time later on the city streets, slurping something from a can, a paper wrapper round their cheeks as they crammed in a gargantuan sandwich. They didn't miss lunch. They were just too scared of their reputations as hard men to be seen eating it.

Always stop for lunch. People often complain that they don't have time for lunch, but that is putting yourself and your physical needs second, or even third, in your priorities, and you mustn't do that.

Lunch is a light meal, high in fibre and water content – these are the most important weapons against cellulite. You have two main choices for lunch, the Cellulite Buster Big Salad or cottage cheese and fruit salad. The basic Big Salad has a list of protein additions which you can rotate according to your mood. You'll can assemble the basic ingredients at the weekend, and then simply scoop out your lunch serving every day. It is an easy meal to transport in snap-shut containers to eat at work, on a train, in the park or, of course, you can eat it at home in the usual way. Cottage cheese and fruit salad works in the same way and, as you will have had a good breakfast, this meal simply keeps you going for those few hours in the afternoon and early evening before you have dinner, without burdening you with calories or indigestible fats and sugars. You won't get the 4 o'clock slumps with a Big Salad!

Make sure you drink at least a large glass of water as well as your normal tea or coffee or whatever you like to have with lunch. But you won't feel hungry because of your substantial breakfast and the promise of dinner. Don't munch on something while continuing to work.

Dinner

Dinner is your re-fuelling meal. Your stocks of fuel are kept in your muscles, primed for the next bit of action. At the end of the day your stocks are empty, like the supermarket shelves after a busy Saturday. Eating now will re-stock, just as a delivery in the supermarket will go straight to the shelves, not the storeroom. You might be relaxing, but while you catch up on the TV programmes, your body is re-fuelling as fast as it can. It has to see you through the evening and right through the night, and waking in the night is often a sign that you didn't re-stock properly, with a good, mixed carbohydrate and protein meal.

Your dinner isn't massive, but it is substantial. You can eat potatoes at this meal if you choose. If you prefer other starchy vegetables, fine, and if you can go through the night without needing extra carbohydrate fine too. When you get to Phase Two you'll find it still allows for some potatoes, but it's up to you whether you have them or not. Dinner will also contain one very high protein element, such as salmon or chicken. Sugar and sweet desserts are completely banned, but there's a pleasant surprise in the addition of a cheese course.

Dinner has two courses as you would expect, but there are three options:

— savoury starter and main course
— main course and pudding
— main course and savoury afters with an optional extra dessert
  course for special occasions or waning willpower!

Making every meal count

If you are going to be successful, slim and glamorous for ever, you have to take this rule seriously. It's not just the food you ate that made you fat – it's the food you forgot you ate; it's the food you never even tasted. The mint from someone's desk, the dipping of the fork into someone else's meal just to have a taste. The bite of a sandwich. Eating at your desk, eating standing in the kitchen, eating while you drive your car – the list goes on. These are not just death to your diet; they're really bad habits.

You're only human and it's easy to be tempted, but really it's hardly worth eating these things. Next time you find yourself having a bite or a mouthful, count 50 calories. It might be more or it might be less, but count 50 anyway. You'd be amazed how this mounts up, and at the end of a day it could be six mouthfuls – that's not just 300 calories today but 2,100 calories a week or 9,000 in thirty days. Nine thousand calories is over a kilo. So when you say that you can't understand why your weight is creeping up, is this maybe a clue? And it's not as if they were enjoyable, memorable meals!

Make your meals count. Respect your body. Sit down and slow down. Your body will thank you for it.

A clean mouth

This is a bit of a trick. It is vital to put a 'full stop' to your eating time with a clean mouth. Just as you would clear the table and wash up, it's really important to clean your teeth, floss and rinse out with warm water. You may already do this – and if you do, great. We've been told that eating a piece of fruit or cheese cleans the teeth after a meal, but what I'm really after is a way of removing the taste of food altogether. It's not a nice thing to say but people leave a lot of food debris in their mouths. In crevices under the lips and at the corners near the wisdom teeth. Not only does this cause bad breath, it's a constant reminder of food. Take away the taste with a good rinse. It does your teeth a favour, prevents plaque build-up and freshens the breath. It also prevents you picking at food. People rarely want to spoil their clean mouths by having another bite of something, so if you don't do it already, carry a fold-up, holiday-type toothbrush in your handbag and maybe a bit of floss.

Food file

Fibre

Fibre is in plant foods. Anything that is a leaf or a fruit, a nut or a root, a seed or a bean, has fibre. Some foods have more fibre than others. You need about 20g fibre per day, which sounds like it's easy to get, but note that the values I've given in the table opposite are per 100g.

If you were to ask me what is the single most neglected element in modern diets, I'd say it was fibre. We are also often dangerously low in iron, but a few days of an iron-rich diet and supplements and we're back to normal: a lack of fibre leads to all sorts of nasty illnesses that have extremely unpleasant side effects. Modern diets are to blame because the process of refining things like wheat flour and rice, not to mention producing those ghastly industrial oven chips which hardly bear any relation to a potato, has taken all the fibre out of these wonderful healthy foods. With nothing for our stomachs to work on, they slide through your system like sludge. They cause something called 'delayed gastric emptying'. It's not the most elegant topic, but it's one you have to be familiar with if you're going to rid your body of toxins, get a flatter stomach and banish those fluid-filled, fat-filled cells that are cellulite.

Gastric emptying

It's not very charming, but it's a topic I've got to mention. Delayed gastric emptying is one of the main causes of excess fat and cellulite. It's like a blocked sink. Lack of fluid to flush things through makes matters a lot worse, so this is a detoxification diet in the true sense. It's HIGH in soluble fibre and LOW in refined carbohydrates.

Chew a low-fat mouthful of crisps and you'll see what I mean. A ball of pulp. Your calorie-counted ready meal with white rice also becomes a mushy mass inside you. This is what is slowing down your gut emptying time, causing a build-up of old food in your digestive system, making you bloated and tired and causing fat deposits on your inactive bits like legs and bottom – and giving you cellulite!

Fibre values

The table below shows the fibre content of foods in grammes per 100 g.

g	Vegetables	g	Pulses		Fruit (cont.)	g	Cereals
3	broccoli	16	kidney beans	1	peaches	1	rice
2	cabbage	16	butter beans	1	pineapples	7	oatmeal
4	Brussels sprouts	28	broad beans	7	prunes (dried)	1	rolled (porridge)
2	cauliflower	11	chick peas	6	prunes (ready		oats
2	turnips	16	soya beans (dried)		to eat)	1	corn (fresh)
3	red cabbage	5	peas	2	prunes (canned)		
4	artichokes	5	lentils	2	pears	g	Bread
2	asparagus			22	figs (fresh)	2	white
1	celery			8	figs (dried)	4	brown
1	pumpkins	g	Salad greens	3	cranberries	6	wholemeal
2	butternut squash	1	lettuce	2	raisins	2	pitta
2	acorn squash	2	spinach	1	strawberries	4	rye
1	courgettes	1	watercress	1	grapes	2	naan
1	marrow	2	endive	4	blackcurrants		
		1	chicory	3	blackberries	g	Nuts
	Root	1	cress	2	blueberries	7	almonds
g	vegetables	1	tomatoes	2	gooseberries	4	Brazils
2	carrot	1	spring onions	3	loganberries	4	chestnuts
2	beetroot	2	peppers	3	redcurrants	7	coconut
2	turnip		(red/green/yellow)	3	raspberries	7	hazelnuts
2	swede			2	oranges	3	cashews
1	radishes	g	Fruit	1	grapefruit	5	pecans
5	parsnip	2	apples	4	kumquats	6	peanuts
1	new potato	2	apricots	1	tangerines	6	pistachios
2	sweet potato	3	avocado	2	papaya	4	walnuts
		1	bananas	3	mango		

Carbohydrates

There's a lot of talk about low-carbohydrate diets, but I'm not in favour of them. I learned to love a hearty bowl of breakfast porridge and an energy-packed lunch of pasta when I was pregnant and had to endure a long bus journey and a thirty-minute walk to the hospital with a young toddler in tow, then an interminable wait and a two-hour trek back home again to fill up the coal scuttle and set about an hour's hand washing. I needed the energy! Contrast this with getting the car out of the garage, loading the washing machine and coming home to pop a few cartons in the microwave. The calorie difference, on top of the sheer effort of keeping warm in a non-centrally-heated house, must have run into thousands every week. And I did this for years.

So there are carbohydrates and carbohydrates. The heavy, starchy carbohydrates like bread, pasta and potatoes are important if you have a gruelling day because they pack a good calorie punch without clogging fats or sugars. But if you don't have this sort of day, avoid them and have lighter carbohydrates instead, like fruit, vegetables and dairy products which are satisfying without providing as much energy (calories). You might have thought that milk was purely a protein food with a variable amount of fat, but it is also a carbohydrate, and half a pint of milk supplies a little less carbohydrate than a banana. A glass of milk provides an instant snack with plenty of brain-dependent glucose, but without the bulk or digestive demands of the banana. It's your choice, but cellulite busting depends on limiting calories from all sources, so I'd recommend sticking with light carbohydrates, and saving bread and potatoes for your main meals.

Proteins

The recent advice about high-protein diets is confusing. It suggests that by cutting carbohydrates to very low levels and increasing protein, you are somehow cutting calories, but this is not the case. Protein is essential for the human processes of growth, maintenance and repair of tissue, hair, nails, etc., but it isn't a magical formula for weight loss. Carbohydrates can have far fewer calories than protein. A salmon fillet has 300 calories whereas a jacket potato has 200 calories. So which is better for you? The answer is that no food is good or bad in itself, and if you had eaten salmon every day for a week your body would need the nutrients in the potato. If you ate potatoes for seven days, a nice salmon fillet would redress the balance. One food item, or one diet element, like protein, cannot make your diet either good or bad or make you lose or gain weight. So keep up daily protein portions, but do not let popular myths like high-protein, low-carbohydrate diets fool you into believing that they are some kind of magic pill for weight loss.

Proteins should be 'nutrient dense'. That means you get a lot in a small package. Say you need 50g of protein a day, to get that amount from carbohydrates you would have to eat 16 slices of bread or 7 jacket potatoes. A piece of fish the size of a playing card provides our entire day's requirement of quality protein, so proteins from animal sources are the only ones which are called 'complete' proteins.

Protein is the nutrient responsible for the repair, maintenance and growth of every bit of your body. If you ate a completely carbohydrate diet without protein you would eventually start wasting. However, too much protein causes fluid loss, kidney stones and even gout. You need to eat about 1g of protein for every kilogram of your body weight (2g if you are a bodybuilder, 3–4 g if you are disabled or elderly. Here are some examples of protein values:

Food	Protein (g)	Food	Protein (g)
150g fillet steak	45.0	boiled egg	6.3
150g chicken breast	25.0	2 tbsp broad beans	9.5
150g tuna or salmon	25.0	150g baked potato	7.0
40g oat-based muesli	5.3	30g porridge oats	4.0
2 slices granary bread	6.0	120g plain live yogurt	7.0
120g cottage cheese	15.0	2 tbsp chick peas	25.0
50g Brie	8.0	3 tbsp peas	4.2
6 walnuts	3.0	corn on the cob	3.2
300ml skimmed milk	9.7		

Fats

Heard the one about fat making you fat? How could it? Since when did you drink double cream or stick a piece of butter on your plate and eat it with a knife and fork? Fats are divided into those in food (meat, chicken, cheese) and those that need something else to go with them (oil, butter).

It's hard to eat too much fat if you take away the things they go with. If you don't eat scones or snacky toast or rogue sandwiches, what would you do with that butter?

Animal fat is a bit of a bad boy but again, there's no problem if you don't go mad. A steak, eggs, a milkshake and three slices of toast and butter, while perfectly healthy individually, are pushing your health luck a bit far if you eat them all in the same day. Animal fats are the artery-clogging fats that kill, but don't get rid of them, limit them.

Good fats are the polyunsaturates and monounsaturates. They are found in foods such as olive oil, avocados, nuts and fish. Oils are quite high in calories, but as long as you watch the amount you use your diet will really benefit from them.

The general advice is that an adult woman should have an intake of 70g of fat a day, but this is a blanket figure for all fats. Personally I only ever look at the saturated fat content of a product, and a top limit of 21g is about right. Here are some saturated fat values of foods you'll find in this diet:

Food	Saturated fat (g)	Food	Saturated fat (g)
30g Brie	7.0	200g fillet steak	7.4
6 walnuts	1.0	300ml skimmed milk	0.3
150g salmon fillet	2.5	One boiled egg	1.5
150g chicken breast	1.2		

So you see, it isn't as scary as it seems to eat eggs and nuts. It makes sense not to eat too many animal products on the same day, but as hardly anyone eats steak breakfasts these days, I think you'll find that by following my method, the fat limits itself.

Fluids

It is important to take a *lot* of fluid on this diet. This includes fluids you drink and fluids that are in your food. All food has water in it. Even bread or meat contain water, and of course fruit and vegetables have the most. A third of your daily intake of fluid comes from your food, which is one reason why people get headaches when they go on a crash diet or starve themselves because you are depriving yourself of glucose (for the brain to work properly) and water.

You must drink plain water on this diet, and rather than suggest alarming amounts like two large bottles a day, I advise you to go for frequent sips instead. This just makes it easier to tolerate. Water isn't the most exciting drink in the world and to be honest, I have to force myself to drink it. But I do! As with all the advice in this book, my method is to do the things that are good for you and you'll get used to them. Try not to drink too much water with your meals and drink most of your water between meals. Fluids dilute stomach acid and that can impair digestion, leading to bloating. You need good amounts of acid for digestion – but if you like drinking water with your meals and don't have a problem with bloating, carry on.

Recommended	Only Phase Two	Banned
plain water	wine (4 or 5 times a week)	fruit-flavoured water
herbal/fruit tea		full-caffeinated coffee/tea
vegetable juices (such as V8)	decaffeinated coffee/tea (only with breakfast)	sweetened fruit juices or squashes
fresh fruit juices		

So what am I going to eat?

Your key foods are:

— fish
— high-fibre vegetables
— bananas, berries and stoned fruits
— nuts and seeds

Fish is important in the Cellulite Buster Diet, and vegans who do not eat any high-protein fish or dairy foods might find themselves not suited to this diet (see page 56).

Fish

Fish should be eaten several times a week. There is so much fish to choose from, you won't get sick of it. It has so many wonderful properties, and you get an awful lot of protein packed into a tiny portion. You would have to eat seven platefuls of peas to get the same amount of protein contained in one small fillet of salmon.

The table opposite shows the nutrients contained in a 100g of various fish.

Fish has other benefits:

— It won't make you bloated.
— It is good for delicate digestions.
— It is quick and easy to cook.
— One piece gives you nearly a full day's quota of protein (depending on your size).
— The beauty advantages are vast – fish helps hair, skin and nails to grow as they've never grown before!

Being good for the digestion is one of fish's most appealing attributes. Red meat or poultry, while being very good for you, take several

Nutrients per 100g	Protein (g)	Fat (g)	Magnesium (mg)	Zinc (mg)	Selenium (mcg)
Salmon	20	11	32	0.7	31
Kippers	18	18	66	2.5	56
Sardines	25	5	18	0.8	20
Mackerel	19	16	45	1.2	58
Tuna	24	5	30	1	83
Prawns	23	1	49	2	23
Crab	20	6	58	6	17
Scallops	23	1	42	3	51
Lobster	22	2	34	3	130
Mussels	17	3	38	2	43

Nutrients per 100g	Calories	Calcium (mg)	Vitamin D (mcg)	Vitamin E (mg)	Vitamin B12 (mcg)
Salmon	180	21	8	2	4
Kippers	230	53	8	0.3	10
Sardines	195	130	12	0.3	12
Mackerel	220	11	8	0.3	10
Tuna	136	16	7	—	4
Prawns	99	60	—	—	4.8
Crab	128	—	—	—	—
Scallops	118	—	—	—	—
Lobster	103	55	trace	1.3	2.5
Mussels	104	—	—	—	—

hours to digest. Only eat red meat when you are having an early evening meal.

Oily fish v. white fish

Which is better for you – oily fish like salmon or trout or white fish like cod or plaice? And what's the difference?

Oily fish has its oils distributed right through its body, in the flesh you eat, while the oil in white fish is stored in the liver. If you eat cod, plaice, haddock and so on, I recommend that you also take a daily fish-oil capsule.

White fish is extremely low in calories and fat, but it lacks the essential fatty acids found in oily fish like salmon and mackerel, and is therefore less nutritious. It also does not have the same appeal when served cold, (if indeed people do serve cod or haddock cold), compared with salmon or tuna, for example, so in a way it lacks the versatility you need on a diet. Because it tends to be bland, people often cover it in sauces or herby crusts, but I strongly suggest you don't do this. Bring out the flavour of the fish by garnishing with parsley or watercress, or serve it on a bed of peppery mashed carrots with beans and peas.

If you eat salmon, choose the organic variety if possible. Traditionally farmed salmon is often reared these days in gigantic tanks, where it swims around in its own dirt. Organic salmon can be identified easily

Fish

Best	OK	Not recommended	Comments
salmon	cod	All fish is recommended	Do not cook with breadcrumb coating, in batter or with a 'crust' – all fish cooked 'bare' and bought fresh
fresh tuna	plaice		
mackerel	haddock		
prawns	halibut		
crab	tinned tuna		
sardines			
mussels			

because it is paler in colour than the bright red/pink of the intensively reared salmon.

Shellfish are low in calories and rich in protein and minerals.

Always take care to get good quality fish.

High-fibre vegetables

Shells or skins on a vegetable, like those on broad beans or peas, are a particularly good source of fibre. The shell not only goes through your body intact, but the vegetable itself tends to be one of the protein-rich types, which vegetables like broccoli and sprouts aren't. Don't get me wrong; all vegetables are good and all vegetables contain valuable fibre, but I prefer the starchier, shell-coated varieties for general cleansing of the gut.

You should have at least one portion of high-fibre vegetables every day.

Asparagus

I have mentioned asparagus separately from all the other high-fibre vegetables because it has special properties and benefits that are particularly good for cellulite. Asparagus is a natural detoxifier. It is known for its pungent flavour and diuretic properties (it helps remove excess fluids). Obviously a key factor of this diet is to remove and replace fluids constantly, rather than not taking enough fluids in the first place or taking a lot of fluids then having them hanging around because you are harbouring high sodium levels which soaks fluid up like a sponge. Drinking plenty of water, eating high-fluid foods like fruit and vegetables and simultaneously eating diuretic foods such as asparagus and celery will make sure you have a rapid transit time for fluids, and nothing in your system for long.

The key benefits of asparagus are:

— It contains potassium, the trace element which helps maintain a good water balance in your body.
— The active ingredients in asparagus include aspargine, aspargose, chelindonic acid and coniferin which, together with potassium, produce the diuretic effect.

— Just six spears gives you enough folate for a day – vital for the formation of the embryo in women who are pregnant or hoping to be pregnant.
— It is useful in treating high blood pressure.
— It is useful for relieving pre-menstrual bloating.

High-fibre vegetables

Best	OK	Not recommended	Comments
asparagus	carrots		Only eat
celery	spinach		potatoes and
broad beans	swedes		root vegetables for dinner
peas	tomatoes		
sweetcorn	salad greens		
broccoli	parsnips		
potatoes			

Fruit

Bananas

You must have a banana every day for breakfast. Bananas have been out of favour for some time with diet specialists, because they have been thought of as too starchy, with too many calories and a particularly high carbohydrate content of 23g per fruit. (An apple contains 10g carbohydrate.) I think this is nonsense. Breakfast is a main meal and you need carbohydrate at this time.

Bananas have a particular benefit: they are very high in potassium. An apple has 120mg potassium, grapes have 210mg and a kiwi fruit 174mg. A banana has a whacking 400mg, only matched by a slice of honeydew melon at 420mg and by avocado pear with 338mg. Bananas also have useful fibre at 3g per fruit, so all in all I have put these high on the list of must have foods.

Low sugar and high potassium

You might think that fruit is so good, you can cram in as much as you like and never get fat. But there is no such thing as a healthy food – just a healthy diet. Whereas I would tell you to eat as many vegetables as you want, I know that you're unlikely to take me at my word and start carrying sneaky containers of steamed carrots and spinach around with you. But apples, pears and grapes are all fruits which we carry with us for when we're stuck in traffic or waiting for a train and, unlike vegetables, they all contain a lot of sugar and therefore can contribute a large amount of carbohydrate and calories. An apple has 50 calories, whereas a tomato has only 10 and a carrot about 20. Enough said.

To deal with cellulite you must eat fruit that is high in potassium and low in sugar. All fruit is good, but cherries and plums have a low glycaemic index and a high potassium content. In fact, all fruits that have a stone are high in potassium with the exception of mangoes, and melon, nectarines and papaya are particularly high in natural sugar. I have included melon as an option for a starter with ham because it is very high in potassium and about 95 per cent water. Potassium regulates your body's water balance. I can't tell you how important this is for beating cellulite. Excess, retained water not only gives you headaches and harbours concentrated waste products but it sits in your tissues, not plumping them up nicely but bogging them down. And where does anything sit? Right where it doesn't get disturbed; on your bottom!

Don't forget prunes either. They occasionally get a bad press because they are high in sugar and calories, but we all know what a fabulous help they are if you are a bit constipated, and of course breakfast is a main meal when calories don't matter as much as at other meals. Do have prunes if your stomach can take them.

Other brilliant fruits are berries of all types. Blueberries, raspberries, blackberries – just ask yourself if berry is in the name and you're home and dry. Blackcurrants, although a wonderful fruit with a high-fibre coating, unfortunately have to have sugar on them when stewing because they are so tart without it, but try to use as little sugar as possible. The vitamin C content of blackcurrants is so ridiculously high, I suggest you grab as many as you can when they are in season. Another good way to get them is in those supermarket bags they call Fruits of the Forest.

They usually have redcurrants and blackberries too, making it a brilliant, cellulite-busting topping for yoghurt.

Potatoes

Potatoes are a good source of potassium and vitamin C, but have had a bad reputation for some years for their high starch content. They also have a high glycaemic index, meaning that a potato will raise your blood sugar (glucose) levels quickly. Peeled, boiled new potatoes are the lowest in this category, while baked potatoes with the skin on preserve more of the vitamin C. You will be getting a lot of vitamin C on this diet, and to give you an idea of the vitamin C content, a portion of new potatoes has about 16mg, a portion of red cabbage has 50mg, two tablespoons of broad beans have 10mg, but a portion of blackcurrants gives you a thumping 160mg! Given that an adult woman's total daily intake should be around 40mg, it is rare for someone to be seriously deficient in this vitamin these days. Your daily Cellulite Buster Salad will give you all the vitamins you require, and potatoes are really included in the diet for their energy factor.

Here's how to get the most from potatoes:

— Eat small, boiled new potatoes, if possible. Where I have suggested a small jacket potato, make sure it doesn't weigh more than 100g.
— Only eat potatoes in the evening or at your main meal when you need to switch off and relax (if you are a nightworker this might be in the morning).
— Always eat potatoes with a protein food, like fish, eggs or chicken.

Nuts

Nuts are not fattening! Nuts are wonderful, fabulous powerhouses of nutrition. Like any food that you eat too much of, nuts will contribute to weight gain if you can't stop nibbling them. I have used them as a dessert course with pieces of fruit, so you can choose this on its own if you like, or have it after a cheese course if your appetite demands it. Nuts are a lovely way to end a meal, and they have a lot of fibre. Never snack on nuts – have them as part of a meal.

Nuts

Best	OK	Not recommended	Comments
brazils	pistachios	cashews	Should be added
almonds		salted peanuts	to cereals or as part
walnuts			of a dessert with
			fresh fruit or cheese

ADDITIONAL KEY FOODS

Additional key foods are:

— chicken and turkey
— eggs
— bread
— oats

Chicken and turkey

These wonderful low-fat, light meats are protein rich, easy on the digestion and extremely versatile. Although fish is my main choice because of the wonderful oils it contains, poultry has a good supply of B vitamins and protein.

Eggs

Forget the scares. Eggs contain cysteine, an amino acid which is present in hair which helps its growth and condition. They also contain B vitamins and have only around 90 calories each for a large egg. Always eat large eggs if you can and try to get organic ones. I am lucky enough to have a few chickens scratching round the garden, and once you have seen and tasted a proper egg you won't want a supermarket one. The yolk is extremely bright yellow due to the grass the hens eat, and provides you with beta carotene. But don't worry if you can only get standard eggs, they're also good. Eggs are the basis of so many quick meals, so include them at least two or three times a week.

Bread

Here's an early morning treat that you'll think about when you go to bed, and dream about while you sleep. You can eat as much bread as you like with your breakfast, but not at any other time of the day. There are no limits, except the type of bread you eat and what you can put on it.

Here are my suggestions:

Wholegrain or multigrain bread

Be very careful about this, as standard supermarket varieties contain flour improving agents, soya flour and additives that help the keeping qualities and freshness of the loaf. Don't touch these! Choose organic loaves from traditional bakeries, or make your own. My recipes for bread (see pages 151–3) are really easy.

Apricot and brazil nut bread

Stores are starting to sell this, but making your own in large batches will ensure a long-lasting supply.

Pumpernickel bread

I once worked in Germany and was astounded by the trim figures of the other young staff who shared my quarters. They always tucked into a good breakfast of German rye bread (pumpernickel) which I thought the vilest-tasting bread imaginable. However, there was nothing else on offer so I had to grit my teeth and eat what I could. I soon realized why Germans favour a range of cold meats and cheeses for breakfast, because these go with pumpernickel quite beautifully and I became a convert, loading my slices of this dark brown nutty bread with tomatoes and cucumber, on top of a little cream cheese, or spreading it with fresh fruit, jam or sliced banana and cottage cheese.

In the evening, the Germans also tended to go for a cold table, and pumpernickel came out again. I stayed in Germany for six months and came home, to the gasps of admiration from my friends, 3 kilos lighter.

Crispbread

If you prefer a lighter breakfast, have crispbread. Multigrain or sesame seed are two of the best, or go for the currant varieties. Again, you may have as much as you like, but only within an hour of waking.

Bread

Best	OK	Not recommended	Comments
home-made multigrain	pitta bread	croissants	Be extra careful about bought breads which boast healthy qualities – most contain soya flour and flour improvers
home-made wheatmeal		brioche	
rye bread		naan	
pumpernickel		crumpets	
rye crispbread		white sliced	
fruit and nut bread		baguettes	
		bloomers	
		burger buns	
		poppy seed rolls	

BANNED FOODS

The dreaded salt

Salt, sodium chloride, is made up of 60 per cent sodium and 40 per cent chloride, and it's the sodium part that matters to us. Every cell in your body needs sodium to work properly: it is essential for the healthy function of nerves and muscles – including your heart muscle – and some nutrients can't be absorbed properly without it. The minimum daily amount you need is 1.6g sodium which is found in about 4g of salt. This is just short of a level teaspoon, which holds 5g. Most people eat far more salt than they need, about 9g a day (two teaspoons) against recommendations by the World Health Organisation that we eat 6g (just over one teaspoon).

Sodium is bad for you because it helps your body to retain fluid. There is a self-regulating system in the body which helps to balance out fluids, but sometimes we override this without realizing it. For example, sweating because we are hot or because we have just done two hours of running or aerobics, results in a large loss of body fluid and our lack of water is signalled by an efficient, recognizable alarm system – being thirsty. But the opposite doesn't really work. Retaining water isn't life-threatening, so your body sees no reason to let you know about it. You simply feel bloated and sometimes quite tired and 'off' and you might have a headache.

Too little fluid, by the way, causes its own problems. This happens when people try to lose weight with diuretic or water pills. They simply force all the available fluid out of their bodies leaving them weak, disorientated, numbed and dehydrated – which is totally counter-productive. Your body is perfectly able to sort its fluid balance out for itself, but just take care not to influence it by having too much salt!

While I have emphasized the need for a lot of extra water in your diet, the idea is for this to pass through your system quickly, flushing through and taking with it any impurities. A normal amount of salt (sodium) in your diet is necessary and your body deals with this in the usual way. The main thing is not to add to your salt intake by eating salted foods, for example:

- tinned soups
- tinned vegetables that do not say 'reduced salt' or 'no added salt'
- some breakfast cereals
- most ready-made meals
- crisps
- salted nuts
- some tinned fish

Look at the labels. Salt is already added to many of the foods you buy, such as some tinned vegetables, baked beans and so on. It is a nuisance to have to trawl through the shelves looking for salt-free products, but you must. Under the ingredients for some tinned sweetcorn, for example, it says 'sweetcorn, sugar, salt'. Don't touch it! There are plenty of other brands on the shelves that have only sweetcorn in them with nothing added, and anyway once you know which brand you like you won't have to think about it again. You are worth this effort.

A word about cheese

This is a recommended food in the diet. Although cheese is high in sodium, it is dependent on the size of the portion. The cheese portions given in the diet are extremely small. As you are getting rid of all the really bad foods in your life, especially processed meals and canned food, you will have more than enough room in your diet for cheese.

Chemicals

Keeping an eye on the number of chemicals in your diet is a good idea.

Chemicals are additives which include preservatives, caking agents, emulsifiers, colourings and flavourings, and a lot more besides. They have to be declared, but who reads every label? Products can sound amazingly friendly and healthy. Take a packet of chicken pieces I bought completely at random from the supermarket, and which could have been the model of complete nutrition for all I knew. I have to admit I was astonished when I read the back of the packet. On the front it simply declared: 'Skinless and boneless chicken. 2 breast fillets.' And then in small italics 'in a light crispy crumb'.

Let me tell you what this contained. Chicken was 62 per cent of the whole, followed by vegetable oil. So far, so good. Then you have:

wheat flour
yeast emulsifier E472
flour treatment agent
ascorbic acid
dextrose
dried skimmed milk
water
modified wheat starch
potato starch
dried egg
raising agent E450
spices and herbs
colours E100, E160
salt
flavouring

So you have the one wholesome ingredient, chicken, and fifteen other ingredients to make your light, crispy crumb. And you wondered why you sometimes feel bloated and uncomfortable?

I don't think we have seen the full effects of this chemical overload in our systems simply because chemicals haven't been around long enough for us to know their real damage potential. It's true to say that in the past tinned products used to have their fair share of additives, but as most people then ate mainly fresh food with a smattering of tinned goods, or a takeaway used to be plain fried fish and chips, I don't think we'll see the real effect of today's diets for another few decades. But we will!

Basically, anything that enters your system which isn't straight-forward food, which your body recognizes, will put you under stress. Smoking stresses your system. It is an attack. Your body is perfectly well able to cope with an attack of pollutants and it mounts its own defence, but forcing it to defend itself on a daily or even hourly basis by smoking, drinking, overloading your system with food, sunbathing and living in a polluted city is asking those defences to work constantly, without rest. All this is serious.

What happens if those cells get overworked? Inside every cell are electrons which like to go round in pairs. Stress forces them to split from their twin and as a result they go round raiding every other cell, splitting them apart to find an electron to pair up with. Now all this sounds a bit far-fetched, but it is what happens and the result is a dead cell. Not so terrible you might think because cells die with the ageing process anyway. But these roaming electrons, which are known as free radicals, are the reason people who smoke, drink a lot of alcohol, or sunbathe frequently and for long periods look older more quickly than people who don't do these things. Free radicals cause most of the damage to your skin and can cause other nasties like cancer.

Cellulite, I am quite convinced, is the result of a constantly stressed system brought about by too much foreign matter in your body; like chemicals and additives in food, too little sleep and too much stress. You feel and look bad. Fresh air, rest and fresh food soon restore your health and your spirits, and the same is true of a diet that gradually gets rid of all these chemicals. Don't eat them!

BUY FRESH FOOD

If you simply can't be bothered checking ingredient labels or get confused or have someone else to do your shopping for you, buy fresh food. You know where you are with fresh food (despite the usual scare stuff about pesticides and moulds – buy organic or give them a good wash!) and you can always be sure that a fresh corn on the cob has no added salt. Carrots or fresh breasts of chicken or a fresh fillet of salmon or cod will have no salt, whereas a ready meal of cod fillet in sauce, while boasting that it contains hardly any calories and that it has an amazing ability to help you shed pounds, probably has far more sodium than you need. The rule has to be that if you have made something yourself, you know what is in it.

However, there is a sting in the tail of the 'natural' claim. Not all natural things are good for you in excess. Manufacturers might boast that something contains only natural ingredients, and of course salt is natural, but then so are deadly nightshade, laburnum seeds and some mushrooms. They could also kill you. I don't want to turn you into a freak who would rather go thirsty than drink tap water or eat that chemical-loaded cake your granny bought for you specially. We are only talking about cellulite, after all! Just be aware, be careful and follow the rules. It is far better to stick to the basic principles of this diet for gradual, lasting improvement and beauty, than go crazy with it and give up exhausted after two months. Be kind to yourself.

YOUR DAY OFF

Sorry to be an old party-pooper, but a day off isn't the green light to eat anything and everything. It shouldn't be the day you look forward to with a glint in your eye and a steely determination to make up for the restrictions of the week with a good blow-out. There would hardly have been any point in having a diet. The Cellulite Buster Diet is a chance to change for the better. With my method of slimming, your day off is simply another way of balancing your diet.

Bodybuilders do this all the time. They have the most restrictive diet imaginable for six days a week but, fanatical though they are, they rest and relax their strict rules once a week on what they call their 'cheat' day. They might eat a high-sodium food like bacon (normally treated like poison), or have custard on their fruit. The difference between a bodybuilder and a true diet die-hard is that the bodybuilder knows he or she is on a regime for the good of his sport. The die-hard does it as a philosophy, so there are no days off. If you are on this diet as a regime with a goal in sight, but still a regime that you intend keeping up for life, you have to have your day off every week. If you don't truly believe in banning chips from your diet, you won't be psychologically robust enough to forget them. So eat them! But only on one day a week.

Here are some suggestions for your day-off diet:

Red meat

Red meat is nutritious, iron- and protein-rich and thanks to modern feeding and rearing methods, lower in fat than some cuts of chicken. On a normal slimming diet I'd recommend red meat at least two or three times a week, but as this is a cellulite busting diet it isn't my top choice. Red meat takes several hours to be fully digested which is why it isn't a good idea for an evening meal, but a fillet, sirloin or rump steak, griddled or barbecued, or a home-made beef casserole in red wine is a delicious treat.

Lamb and pork are other meats you can have on your day off. Minced lamb in particular is brilliant in a lot of exotic dishes like moussaka.

(For vegetarian options, see pages 142–8)

Other 'splurgeworthy' meals

— Dry curries – such as tikka pieces and chicken tandoori, served with plain boiled rice. Allow yourself that poppadum and naan bread.
— Paella and chilli con carne.
— Wholesome quiches and pizzas – don't have thick crusts though.
— Roasts with roast potatoes or chips.
— Fruit cake and oat flapjacks.
— Fruit sorbets and plain ice cream.

Banned foods

Junk food like crisps, ice cream, flavoured yoghurts, low-fat mousses, ready meals or combined items like burgers (which have several components to make the one item) are not allowed, even on your day off. They can't exist without huge numbers of chemicals to bind, texturize and enhance their flavour. They have no place in your body. Cellulite and beautiful legs are not helped by rubbish food and chemicals, so you should aim, throughout this month, to wean yourself off them.

COOKING AND EATING

How to cook and eat your meals is as important as the food itself.

Eat protein first

What do you eat first when you begin a meal? You probably haven't thought about it. Most people get straight to the vegetables and start eating their meat or fish about their third mouthful – I've watched! I'm sure there is some deep psychological behavioural explanation for this, but I like to think that we just want something in our mouths, and we go for the easiest thing! Whatever the reason, my method has a few basic suggestions for getting the most from your meal, and making sure you don't go diving into seconds and thirds too quickly.

Eat your high-quality protein first and this will help damp your appetite more quickly. It sends a message to your brain after a few minutes, which effectively switches off the part that says you're still hungry. If you eat your vegetables first and only get to the protein later, you'll want more.

Keep your food items separate on your plate. You don't have to eat all your protein straight off (this would be incredibly boring!), but do have about half of it before you embark on the vegetables.

Every time you pause to chew, put down your knife and fork. Don't even start cutting the next mouthful before you have swallowed. It's called 'loading your fork' and looks horrible. It's also the reason people get bloated. Digestion starts in the mouth, and if you haven't chewed properly, your stomach won't be in a fit state to deal with it.

Drink a little while you're eating, but try not to wash everything down. Too much water dilutes your stomach acid so it can't digest your food properly. This leads to a feeling of fullness and bloating soon after you've finished eating. Drink plenty of water between meals, but not much during the meal.

Vegetarians

Vegetarians are easily accommodated on the Cellulite Buster Diet, although it is not suitable for vegans as so many of the animal-sourced proteins (dairy, fish) are vital parts of the menus.

Vegetarians can have as many weight and cellulite problems as non-vegetarians. A diet is always only as good as the person who follows it, and quantities of butter, oils, nuts and of course sweets, chocolate and alcohol will turn to excess fat if the calories aren't used as energy. The vegetarian meals on this diet will not have the same variety as non-vegetarian ones, but I have always found that vegetarian friends of mine expect this, and indeed it is no different from any other diet where an entire food group is excluded. However, it is worth reminding ourselves that we have only seven evening meals each week to plan for, and I have never known anyone worry about having something different and exciting for breakfast or lunch every day. Within a non-meat diet there are some wonderful possibilities if you put your mind to it, with the main proviso being that you have variety.

To be sure of variety, you must plan. Now this sounds groaningly time-consuming, but it isn't. Years ago, family meals were predictable. Roast on Sunday, shepherd's pie on Monday, fish on Friday, fry-up on Saturday. I'm not sure what came on the days in between. Each day was different but each day was also predictable. It would be a boring world if we ate the same meal every Monday or Wednesday or whatever, but busy lives need planned menus because lack of planning leads to grabbing whatever food there is to hand – and that leads to a bad diet and weight gain!

Make sure you eat the recommended amount of nuts and seeds for protein, drink skimmed milk and if you like eggs, all the better. With so many vegetables and fruit dishes, you shouldn't find it a problem to really crack your cellulite problem quite easily.

Cooking methods

The cooking on this diet is simple, quick and basic. Your meals are gloriously light and tasty and they look good. I can't see the point of standing over the stove with half a dozen bottles, spices and herbs all over the place, when you can have variety and a tasty meal just by including different textures and combinations of foods. Fish and broccoli, for example, are a lovely combination of crisp and soft; chicken and potatoes the same. So cooking is simplicity itself on your diet.

Although cooking is best done carefully and thoughtfully, it's better to cut corners and eat properly than to give up altogether and opt for a takeaway. Use foil trays and tins which you can buy in hardware stores or supermarkets in the freezer sections and throw them away after you've used them. I get ten for about £1.00, which makes it a cheap throwaway item: after all, it's the scrubbing and scraping of tins and pans which puts us off cooking and encourages us to buy ready meals. You can also just tear off a piece of foil or greaseproof paper and make it up into an 'envelope' for oven baking. Just throw in the ingredients and bake!

Here are the basics:

— Operate the 'one-spare' system. This means that whenever you have to cook one thing, such as a chicken breast or a piece of fish, you cook two instead. The second item is covered and put into the fridge, and you eat it cold the following day.

— Always have a container of peeled and sliced vegetables handy in the fridge. When you have a stir-fry in mind you simply tip them out into the pan. Prepare enough (or buy them ready prepared) for about four meals. There's a school of thought that suggests you lose vitamins by having them ready to eat, but it seems to me that if it comes down to the difference between eating them minus a milligram or two of vitamins because you've sliced them up a couple of days early, and not eating them at all because they're a fuss to prepare, I'd go for the first option!

— The same goes for salads. It only takes ten minutes to assemble everything and keep it in a snap-shut container. If you come home hungry, you could always bring forward your starter by scooping out some salad and tossing it in some vinaigrette. You could add a few broken nuts, some pine nuts or shavings of Parmesan. I don't agree with eating snacks in between meals, but if you're absolutely fainting with hunger and likely to break your diet with a packet of bourbons, it's better to have the salad a bit early.

The Diet: Phase One

— Your day starts with a good breakfast of around 400 calories.
— Your re-fuelling meal in the evening will have between 500–600 calories.
— Your Cellulite Buster Big Salad for lunch has about 250 calories.
— You will then have plenty of calories available for milk in tea and coffee, and extra salads, if necessary.

Breakfast

Breakfast must contain a grain-based food, nuts or seeds, a dairy item and some fruit.

You should have any or most of these to eat for breakfast:

— grains: oats or bread
— nuts and seeds: sprinkled onto muesli or yoghurt
— low-sugar fruits: berries in particular
— high-energy fruit: banana
— a dairy item: plain live yoghurt and skimmed milk
— a non-dairy alternative: soya milk and soya yoghurt
— eggs
— tea or decaffeinated coffee or spring water or water flavoured with fresh orange, lemon or lime slices.

The following breakfast choices are suggestions: feel free to devise your own when you have reached the 'coasting' stage.

Breakfast 1
— 40g porridge (made with water), topped with as much skimmed or soya milk as you choose, no sugar.
— A bowl of sliced banana and mixed berries (blueberries, raspberries, etc., your choice, topped with 1 tbsp plain live yoghurt.

Breakfast 2
— 40g (1 teacup) Cellulite Buster Breakfast Muesli (see recipe below) with a teacupful of skimmed milk.
— Fruit and yoghurt as Breakfast 1.

Breakfast 3
— 2 eggs, cooked any way you choose, 2 slices wholegrain toast.
— Fruit and yoghurt as Breakfast 1.

Breakfast 4
— 2 slices Apricot and Brazil Nut toast (see recipe page 151), with sugar-free orange spread (such as St Dalfour or a supermarket's own brand known as pure fruit preserve with no artificial sweeteners and no added sugar).
— Fruit and yoghurt as Breakfast 1.

Breakfast 5
— Cellulite Buster Protein Shake (see recipe page 147)
— 2 slices multigrain toast with orange spread.

Breakfast 6
— 40g oats soaked overnight or for an hour in a teacupful of soya or skimmed milk, topped with a chopped banana, 1 tsp wheatgerm, 1 tbsp plain live yoghurt and 1 dsp slivered almonds.

Breakfast 7
— A bowl of banana slices, topped with plain live yoghurt and sprinkling with sunflower and pumpkin seeds.
— A boiled egg with a slice of toast thinly spread with butter.

Cellulite Buster Breakfast Muesli

You should find all these ingredients in any health food store.

½ cup toasted wheatgerm (such as Bemax or Froment)
1 cup mixed flaked almonds and broken walnuts
1 cup pumpkin seeds
1 cup sesame seeds
1 cup sunflower seeds
2 cups organic oats
2 cups organic rye flakes

Mix all the ingredients together and put into a tin or snap-shut container. Keep in a cool dry place.

One serving is one cupful.

Lunch

Cellulite Buster Big Salad

This special salad has everything you need and is a main meal with high-protein additions that you can choose to suit yourself. The idea is that it gives you all the important elements in cellulite busting and weight loss, namely fluids, potassium and fibre.

bed of shredded lettuce
handful lamb's lettuce
6 asparagus spears
few sprigs watercress
few rings red pepper
few rings yellow pepper
chicory rings
1 stick celery, chopped
cucumber, finely chopped
carrot, grated
1 dsp sultanas
red or white cabbage, grated

Add any TWO as desired:

½ avocado pear, sliced
1 tbsp pine nuts, toasted
30g cheese, grated
100g tuna fish
1 hard-boiled egg, quartered

Dinner

Dinner is a two-course meal. I have given you six choices for each course – enough for one each day of the week.

Savoury starters

A starter is a good idea. A mixed salad tossed in a nice oily dressing can take the edge right off your appetite, which is important if you've come home ravenous. We often dive into the main course and pile the plate higher than we should simply because we're extra hungry. I've done it myself, but I find that a plate of salad, especially if it has tomatoes and grated carrot which tend to be particularly satisfying, takes the edge right off my appetite. It also stays the hand from dipping into the cereal packet!

There is a soup or salad option for the starter, and I have added corn on the cob as a high-fibre option if you are doing the diet in summer when fresh corn cobs are widely available. You can make the soups yourself if you are handy at this, but no butter or cream must be used – just plain vegetables and beans or lentils, cooked, blended and seasoned. Alternatively, I thoroughly recommend the Covent Garden range of fresh soups or any other brand of fresh soups as long as they have no more than 90 calories per 100ml maximum, and no additives or preservatives.

— corn on the cob
— asparagus, celery, watercress, lentil and bean or vegetable soup
— a mixed salad (plain salad greens, tomato, carrot and celery with vinaigrette) or Waldorf salad

Main courses

200g skinless chicken or turkey breast
200g fillet of salmon
200g white fish
150g tuna fish
150g tofu
150–200g Quorn

PLUS any unlimited amounts of any THREE of these vegetables, eaten without butter or dressings:

asparagus
baby corn
Brussels sprouts

broad beans
broccoli
cabbage
carrots
cauliflower
French beans
mange tout
parsnip
runner beans
spinach
swede

Plus 3 small potatoes, or a small (150g) jacket potato (if you choose).

Cellulite Buster Small Salad

In the summer, you might prefer a side salad with an outdoor meal or a barbecue, or with a cold meal on a hot evening. This is where I recommend the special Cellulite Buster Small Salad, which goes well with hot or cold chicken, grilled steaks or any other protein items. Your usual lunch is, of course, the Cellulite Buster Big Salad, but on weekends, days off or on picnics, you might like to take a portion of this Small Salad to accompany cold meats, eggs or fish, as it is easy to make up and transport.

Basically, it is a salad made from cooked or tinned high-fibre vegetables. Conventional salads have healthy greens in them which are not naturally high in fibre, so my Small Salad is a bit different. I recommend that you make up a bowl of this so it is handy, and the quantities in this recipe will last for about three days for one person.

    12 fresh asparagus spears (a small tin of asparagus, drained, will do)
    12 dsp cooked peas
    12 dsp sweetcorn (buy the no added salt variety)
    3 sticks celery, chopped finely

To assemble, put half an inch of water into a pan and bring to a rapid boil. Add the asparagus spears and cover the pan tightly. Steam on a high boil for 2 minutes, remove and drain. Cool quickly and chop into 2cm pieces, including the stems. Mix with the peas, sweetcorn and celery, cover and keep in the fridge until needed.

Dressings and condiments

I'm mad about oil dressings. Portion sizes should be controlled to a maximum of 2 tablespoons per meal. Recommended dressings are:

— olive oil and vinegar – make it yourself with 2 parts oil to 1 part vinegar and 1 tsp English mustard. A serving is 2 tbsp.
— walnut oil and vinegar – as above but using walnut oil.
— fresh mayonnaise – either make it yourself or buy the variety called 'fresh mayonnaise' found in supermarket chilled salad cabinets. A serving is 2 tsp.
— half-fat crème fraiche – 1 dsp added to chicken or fish in cooking, or mixed with herbs such as dill as a dressing for cold fish.

Dessert course

Your dessert must be fruit based. If you have this meal in the evening, it is a good idea to have your highest-fibre fruit and vegetables now, as they can be processed by your body to better effect when you are asleep.

I have not given exact quantities for these desserts. The basic rule is that you have one portion and can't go back for more, so to some extent this is self-limiting. If this diet allowed, say, four small meals a day, I would suggest very small portions, but this is a main meal dessert and you need nourishment.

Please be sensible. A modest bowl of apple and blackberry with yoghurt is about 150 calories; a massive bowl is 300 calories! The more you eat the more calories you ingest, so in the end you are only hurting yourself if you overindulge.

Eat from a small bowl and don't add sugar. Berries, fresh apricots, plums and cherries are extremely low in calories, while a baked apple with sultanas or stewed apple and blackberries are slightly higher calorie. Fruit is always good for you, so don't stint yourself and enjoy it.

Here are some dessert suggestions:

— apple and blackberry with 1 tbsp plain live yoghurt
— baked apple with or without sultanas
— baked peaches
— baked fresh apricots

— baked peach with or without sherry
— bowl of plums with 1 tbsp plain live yoghurt
— cherries and plums eaten fresh (any amount)
— fresh apricots with 1 tbsp plain live yoghurt
— fresh raspberries with blueberries and 1 tbsp half-fat crème fraiche
— fresh strawberries with 1 tbsp half-fat crème fraiche or plain live yoghurt
— peach slices with blueberries, cherries and kirsch
— plain stewed apple and 1 tbsp half-fat crème fraiche
— winter fruit salad (see page 149)

Cheese course

You should not have any bread, crackers, crispbreads or breadsticks with this course. Basically you may choose a 28g piece of any cheese. This works out roughly as one of those small, individually wrapped portions you might find in supermarket pick'n'mix sections, or if you can trust yourself, buy a larger piece of cheese, cut it into 28g pieces and wrap them individually.

Choose from one of the following:

— 28g cheese, 2 sticks celery, one peach
— 28g cheese, 2 sticks celery, 10 cherries and 6 walnuts
— 28g cheese, 2 sticks celery, 2 fresh apricots
— 28g cheese, 2 sticks celery, 1 apricot and 6 whole almonds
— 28g cheese, 2 sticks celery, 2 plums

The diet

— I have given you exercises to do each day which you can find on pages 118–22.

— You are allowed potatoes at dinner, but monitor yourself carefully. If you have been active and feel you need them, fine. If you have had a particularly lazy day leave them out.

— These menus are all suggestions. Feel free to devise your own menus.

— Do not mix and match within the days, but you may choose any day you like and follow it through, and you may repeat days as often as you like if you find the meals suit you.

— For dinner you may choose either a starter and main course, a main course and dessert or a main and a savoury course.

Breakfast 40g porridge made with water and topped with as much skimmed or soya milk as you like but no sugar
A bowl of 2 dsp mixed berries, 1/2 banana and 1 tbsp plain live yogurt

Lunch Cellulite Buster Big Salad (see page 61)
A few cherries or 3 plums

Dinner *Starter* – Corn on the cob
Main course – Grilled Chicken in Orange Marinade (see page 138), served on a bed of stir-fried vegetables
or – Pan-fried Salmon and Green Lentils with Cellulite Buster Small Salad (see pages 133 and 63)

Dessert Strawberries with 1 tbsp plain live yoghurt, or 1 tbsp low-fat fromage frais or 1 tbsp half-fat crème fraiche

Savoury 28g low-fat soft cheese, 2 sticks of celery, and either 2 plums, 2 fresh apricots or an orange

Exercise 30-minute walk
Your choice of buster block
Full programme of toning exercises

Presentation Full cleansing routine with salt scrub (see page 123)

Breakfast 2 eggs, cooked any way you choose, 2 slices of wholegrain toast
Fruit and yogurt as Day 1

Lunch Cellulite Buster Big Salad (see page 61)
Small bowl of 8 whole almonds and 1 dsp raisins

Dinner *Starter* – 250ml bowl soup (for choice see list on page 62)
Main course – Plain poached or pan-fried salmon with Cellulite
Buster Small Salad (see pages 63 and 132)
or – Lentil Salad but include mixed beans, pine nuts and walnut
oil dressing (see pages 138–9)

Dessert Raspberries and blueberries mixed, with 1 tbsp half-fat crème
fraiche, low-fat fromage frais or plain live yoghurt

Savoury 28g Cheddar or Edam, 2 sticks celery, 1 tbsp raisins

Exercise *During the day* – Your choice of buster block plus a 30-minute
walk
In the evening – 100 bottom squeezes
20 all-fours gluteal and hamstring toner
100 bottom squeezes
20 all-fours gluteal and hamstring toner
stretch

Presentation Fake tan (see page 125)

Breakfast   40g (1 teacupful) Cellulite Buster Breakfast Muesli (see page 60) with a teacupful of skimmed or soya milk
Fruit and yogurt as Day 1

Lunch   Cellulite Buster Big Salad (see page 61)
3 plums, handful of cherries or a small serving strawberries

Dinner   *Starter* – Prawn salad: 100g prawns mixed with 1 tsp mayonnaise (see page 64), served on a bed of shredded lettuce and watercress
Main course – Barbecued or plain oven-roasted chicken breast with 2 potatoes and two other green vegetables or Cellulite Buster Small Salad
or – Vegetable Kebabs with Salsa (see page 144) and a jacket potato

Dessert   Strawberry, Banana and Peach Kebab (see page 149)

Savoury   28g cheese, 2 sticks celery, 1 apricot and 6 whole almonds.

Exercise   Your choice of buster block
30-minute walk
Full programme of toning exercises

Presentation   Have a shower and gently massage each leg with soap for 5 minutes. You must be careful not to rub off your tan

DAY 4

Breakfast   2 slices of Apricot and Brazil Nut toast (see page 151) with
                 sugar-free orange spread
                 Fruit and yogurt as Day 1

Lunch   Cellulite Buster Big Salad (see page 61)
                 A peach or a nectarine

Dinner   *Starter* – Corn on the cob
                 Main course – Pan-fried Salmon with Green Lentils (see
                 page 133) and two other vegetables
                 or – Grilled Vegetable Salad with Creamy Dressing (see
                 page 144)

Dessert   Baked Peach in Sherry (see page 150) with 1 tbsp half-fat
                 crème fraiche

Savoury   28g cream cheese with garlic and chives, 2 sticks celery,
                 10 cherries or 10 grapes

Exercise   30-minute power walk
                 Your choice of buster block
                 No toning programme today EXCEPT the stretching exercise

Presentation Massage with oils or cream (see page 125)

Breakfast   40g oats soaked overnight or for at least an hour in a teacupful
                of skimmed or soya milk topped with a chopped banana,
                1 tsp wheatgerm, 1 tbsp plain live yogurt and 1 dsp slivered
                almonds

Lunch   Cellulite Buster Big Salad (see page 61)
                Small bowl of 8 whole almonds and 1 dsp raisins

Dinner   *Starter* – Large mixed salad
                Main course – Poached cod fillet and boiled potatoes with
                broccoli and sprouts or French beans
                or – Baby Spinach, Potato and Egg Salad (see page 143)

Dessert   Bowl of plums with 1 tbsp plain live yoghurt

Savoury   28g cheese, 2 sticks celery, 2 plums or 10 cherries

Exercise   Aerobic video
                Full programme of toning exercises adding in some abdominal
                exercises and repeating the inner thigh sequence one more
                time

Presentation Full body-cleansing routine and leg shaving (see page 124)
                Massage with oil after removing all fake tan

Breakfast	Cellulite Buster Protein Shake (see page 147)
	2 slices Multigrain toast with sugar-free orange spread

Lunch   Cellulite Buster Big Salad (see page 61)

Dinner   *Starter* – 250 ml bowl of soup (for choice see list on page 62)
Main course – Malibu Salad (see page 141) with a jacket potato
    (optional)
or – Large Waldorf Salad (see page 147)

Dessert   Fresh fruit salad made with any three, stoned fruits or mixed
    berries, topped with 1tbsp low-fat fromage frais or 2 tbsp
    half-fat evaporated milk

Savoury   28g cheese, 2 celery sticks, 6 almonds and a peach or an orange

Exercise   Your choice of buster block
    30-minute power walk
    Hip toning lifts – 20 each side
    Side leg lifts – 20 each leg

Presentation   Apply new fake tan (see page 125)

DAY 7

Day off (see page 54)

DAY 8

Breakfast   A bowl of banana slices topped with 1 tbsp plain live yogurt
and sprinkled with sunflower and pumpkin seeds
A boiled egg with one slice of toast thinly spread with butter

Lunch   Cellulite Buster Big Salad (see page 61)
A peach or a nectarine

Dinner   *Starter* – Corn on the cob
Main course – 150g pan-fried tuna steak with boiled, sliced and
pan-fried potatoes and unlimited amounts of two other
vegetables from the list on pages 62–3
or – an unlimited amount of stir-fried vegetables with soy
sauce, served on a bed of 4 tbsp boiled rice

Dessert   Large dish of sliced strawberries topped with 1 tbsp plain live
yoghurt or 2 tbsp half-fat evaporated milk

Savoury   28g cream cheese or 28g Stilton, 2 sticks celery, 10 cherries

Exercise   Your choice of buster block
Full programme of toning exercises
Add in 2 x 20 abdominal crunches today

Presentation   Repeat cleansing programme and application of tan as for days
1–6
Apply new fake tan in the same pattern – scrub off after 4 days,
reapply after 5 days

Breakfast   2 eggs cooked any way you choose, 2 slices of wholegrain toast
Fruit and yoghurt as Day 1

Lunch   Cellulite Buster Big Salad (see page 61)
A bowl of strawberries and blueberries or nectarine and plum
slices

Dinner   *Starter* – A mixed green salad with 1 tbsp Parmesan or Cheddar,
grated or shaved. Serve with 1 dsp of salad dressing (see
list page 64)
Main course – 3-egg Spanish omelette with Cellulite Buster
Small Salad (see page 63) and 3 boiled new potatoes
(optional)
or – Grilled Vegetable Salad with Creamy Dressing (see
page 144), served with mashed potato or 3 tbsp rice

Dessert   Mixed fresh fruit salad, including mango, berries and peach
or – Small ramekin of whole almonds and large sultanas

Savoury   28g cream cheese with fresh apricots and almonds, 2 sticks
celery and 2 plums or an apple

Exercise   Aerobics video
30-minute walk
Full programme of toning exercises

Exercises

Do these exercises *every day* on the Cellulite Buster programme. They take about thirty minutes.

You might want some music to inspire you. You'll have your favourite sounds, but as a guide to tempo, the Diana Ross hit 'Chain Reaction' has the right number of beats per minute (124).

These exercises work your entire thigh and hip area. Starting at the front of your thigh, they travel round using outer thigh, hip and buttock muscles, moving on to hamstrings and inner thighs, all in one smooth programme. You don't need any fancy equipment or exercise aids, although I do recommend the use of a weight of some sort for the final hamstring lifts when you get better at it.

Warm-up first

You should do your aerobic exercise first, or even just go for a walk. If you're really unable to do anything, don't go into these exercises cold – walk up and down stairs six times first, circle your arms a dozen times, bend and straighten your knees twelve times. Have a good stretch!

Top of thigh lifts

1. Sit on the floor as shown, arms straight and palms flat, fingers pointing away from you. Don't slump in the middle – your torso should be dead straight.

2. Stretch both legs out in front and point toes as hard as you can. Lift your left leg.

3. Keeping your knee straight, slightly cross the leg over the lower one, then raise up. Do eight lifts slowly.

4. Now do sixteen lifts at double time. This is hard, and the top of your thigh really feels it. Keep going!

5. Do another eight lifts slowly.

6. Then sixteen lifts at double time.

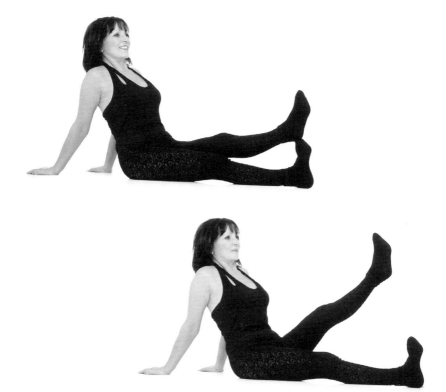

ide leg lifts

Lie on your side, keeping your upper body well away from the floor and supporting it by putting your hand on the floor. Make sure your neck and head don't sink into your shoulder.

Raise and lower your top leg, letting it just touch the floor in front of your lower leg. Do this the same tempo as the last exercise, eight times slowly and sixteen times at double time.

Repeat the set once more.

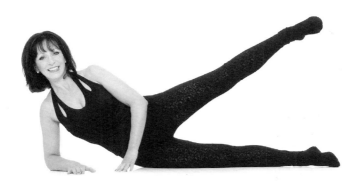

Hip-toning lifts

1. Still lying on your side, shift your top hip forwards, bottom leg backwards, and place your top elbow on the floor. This forces your body right over, as if you were going to lie face down. Take the top leg up and back, dead straight.

2. From the upwards position, lower your leg until your toe just touches the floor behind your other leg. As before, do eight slowly then sixteen at double time, then repeat.

3. Your leg mustn't be raised too high. The important movement is the downwards one, and you need to feel the stretch in your hip as you make this move.

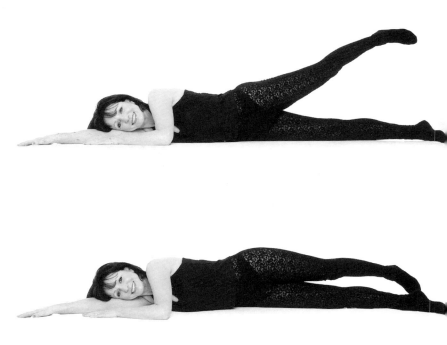

All-fours gluteal and hamstring toner

. Get on your hands and knees and make sure your back and neck are in alignment, and your back isn't dipped in the middle. You should be looking straight down at the floor.

. Stretch out your right leg as shown and hold. Point your toe and concentrate on straightening your knee and stretching your leg as much as possible. Hold your abdomen in tightly.

. Now, flex your foot, then point it, in a 'pulsing' movement. Each time, your leg is raised a few centimetres, and you will feel the effort in your buttocks.

. Do 24 pulses. Rest a few seconds then do another 24 pulses.

. Rest by sitting your bottom back on your heels, stretching your arms forwards and placing your head between your arms.

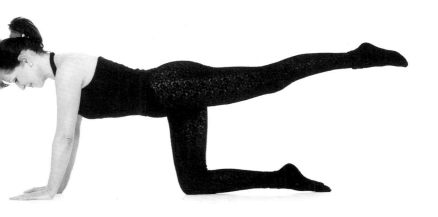

Inner-thigh toner

1. Lie on your back. Place your hands or fists just under your hips as shown. This helps to stop your back arching.

2. Take both legs high and stretch them as wide as you can. (This might not be very wide, but don't worry – it'll come.) Now point your toes hard, and concentrate on making your knees straight. Don't worry if they won't go straight either – they will!

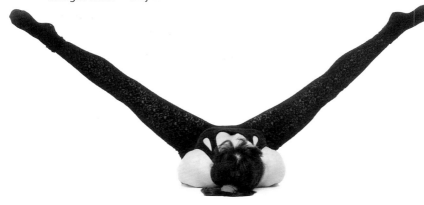

3. You're going to do slow scissoring movements, bringing your feet together and then stretching your legs apart. Try not to let your legs just fall apart – they should be controlled all the time, with your toes still pointed. When your legs get to their farthest point, feel as if you are just elongating that little bit more – s-t-r-e-t-c-h!!

4. Bring your legs together and do tiny scissoring movements. Do eight then let legs fall apart, eight more and stretch and so on – do this as many times as you can. I suggest eight complete repetitions.

5. Bring your knees into your chest and relax.

bottom squeezes

Lay on your back. You can do this as you are or place a weight on your hips. Raise and lower quickly a 100 times, pressing your knees together and releasing each time.

Great! You've gone full circle and are ready to repeat the exercises with your right leg.

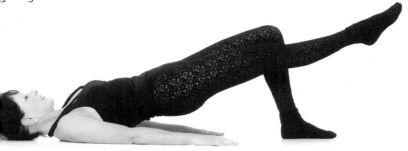

stretch 1

This exercise stretches the whole lower back and outer thigh area.

Sit as shown, gradually lean forwards over your crossed legs as you feel the stretch. Beginners should not worry if they can only go a little way – holding and then increasing the stretch by a few centimetres will soon develop to the full stretch. Make sure you don't force this move!

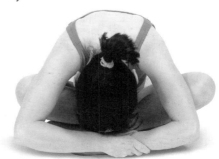

Stretch 2

To stretch backs of legs, all you need is a chair, stool or table. You can do this any time in any clothes, but take off your shoes first. Place both arms on the surface and step backwards. Stand with both feet level, and make sure your stretch is not too wide – your hips should be over your feet.

Try to flatten your back as you lower your head between your arms as I am doing. This is also a good all-round stretch for your back, shoulders and arm.

Stretch 3

This is tough, so take it easy at first. Take position as I am doing. Reach backwards and try to take hold of your opposite foot – i.e. left hand to right foot. This is a string stretch for your thigh and entire hips area and it balances the work you have done on the backs of your legs. Never neglect the fronts of your thighs as they are as important as the backs, and stretching makes them look long and lean.

If you find this difficult, keep your back foot on the floor and simply lean forwards.

Breakfast   2 slices Apricot and Brazil Nut toast (see page 151) with
              sugar-free orange spread
              Fruit and yoghurt as Day 1

Lunch   Cellulite Buster Big Salad (see page 61)
              Strawberries or 3 plums

Dinner   *Starter* – 250ml bowl soup (for choice see list on page 62) or
              mixed crudités with low-fat cottage or cream cheese dip
              (any flavour)
              Main course – Foil-baked salmon with courgettes, fresh dill,
              carrot sticks, served with Cellulite Buster Small Salad (see
              page 63)
              or – Avocado and pine nut salad: 1 avocado, sliced, 1 dsp pine
              nuts, toasted, 1 tbsp salad dressing (see page 64)

Dessert   Peach, Blueberry and Cherry Fruit Salad with Kirsch (optional)
              (see page 148)

Savoury   28g cheese, 2 sticks celery, 1 apricot and 6 whole almonds

Exercise   Your choice of buster block
              30-minute walk
              4 sets of inner thigh exercises
              4 sets of side leg lifts
              4 sets of top of thigh exercises
              4 sets all-fours gluteal and hamstring toner
              4 sets hip toning lifts

Breakfast	2 slices Multigrain toast with sugar-free orange spread *and* Cellulite Buster Protein Shake (see page 147)
Lunch	½ avocado, sliced, with 2 tbsp prawns, served with salad *or* – Cellulite Buster Big Salad (see page 61)
Dinner	*Starter* – Corn on the cob *Main course* – Stir-fried chicken with a large portion of asparagus and courgettes and a small jacket potato (optional) *or* – Baby Spinach, Potato and Egg Salad (see page 143)
Dessert	Bowl of plums with 1 tbsp plain live yoghurt
Savoury	28g hard cheese, 2 sticks celery, 2 fresh apricots
Exercise	30-minute power walk Your choice of buster block No toning programme today EXCEPT the stretching exercise

DAY 12

Breakfast   40g oats soaked overnight or for at least an hour in a teacupful
of skimmed or soya milk topped with a chopped banana,
1 tsp wheatgerm, 1 tbsp plain live yogurt and 1 dsp slivered
almonds

Lunch   Cellulite Buster Big Salad (see page 61)
A fresh peach or in winter tinned peach slices in fruit juice not
syrup

Dinner   *Starter* – 1/2 avocado with salad dressing (see page 64) or
slices of smoked salmon with lemon and capers
Main course – Grilled plaice with mashed carrots, peas and new
potatoes
or – 150g pan-fried tofu with vegetables as above

Dessert   Winter Fruit Salad (see page 149) topped with 1 tbsp plain live
yoghurt

Savoury   28g low-fat cream cheese or Brie with 2 celery sticks and a pear

Exercise   Your choice of buster block
30-minute walk
Full programme of toning exercises

Breakfast	2 eggs, cooked any way you choose, with 2 slices of wholegrain toast
	Fruit and yoghurt as Day 1
Lunch	Cellulite Buster Big Salad (see page 61)
	A few grapes
Dinner	*Starter* – Grated carrot, watercress and sweetcorn salad
	Main course – Chicken, Asparagus and Chickpea Salad (see page 139)
	or – Stir-fried vegetables with 150g tofu cubes and pine nuts
Dessert	4 sliced fresh plums with 1 tbsp half-fat crème fraiche, or, if tinned, 6 whole plums
Savoury	28g cheese, 2 celery sticks, 6 walnuts and a few raisins
Exercise	A yoga or Pilates class if possible
	Walk/run programme
	100 bottom squeezes
	20 all-fours gluteal and hamstring toners
	100 bottom squeezes
	20 all-fours gluteal and hamstring toners
	Stretching exercise

Day off (see page 54)

Breakfast   A bowl of banana slices topped with 1 tbsp plain live yogurt
                and sprinkled with sunflower and pumpkin seeds
                A boiled egg with one slice of toast thinly spread with butter

Lunch   Cellulite Buster Big Salad (see page 61)
                A peach

Dinner   *Starter* – Corn on the cob or a 250ml bowl of lentil soup
                Main course – Salmon with Fruit and Nut Sauce (see page 134)
                or – Basic Pan-fried Vegetables with Parmesan and Pine Nuts
                    (see page 142)

Dessert   Baked Peach in Sherry (see page 150) with 1 dsp half-fat crème
                fraiche or 1 tbsp half-fat evaporated milk

Savoury   28g cheese, 2 sticks celery and 2 plums or an apple

Exercise   Your choice of buster block
                30-minute power walk
                Hip toning lifts – 20 each side
                Side leg lifts – 20 each leg
                Stretching exercise

Breakfast	Cellulite Buster Protein Shake (see page 147)
	2 slices Multigrain toast with sugar-free orange spread
Lunch	Cottage Cheese and Fruit Salad (see page 147)
Dinner	*Starter* – Waldorf Salad (see page 147)
	Main course – Plain roast chicken breast with broccoli, sprouts and carrots. 2 boiled potatoes if you've had an active day
	or – 3-egg cheese omelette with Cellulite Buster Small Salad (see page 63), boiled potatoes (optional)
Dessert	Winter Fruit Salad (see page 149) topped with 1 tbsp plain live yoghurt
	or – Fresh raspberries and 1 tbsp plain live yoghurt
Savoury	28g cheese, 2 sticks celery, 2 fresh apricots
Exercise	30-minute power walk
	Your choice of buster block
	No toning programme today EXCEPT the stretching exercise

Breakfast   40g oats soaked overnight or for at least an hour in a teacupful of skimmed or soya milk topped with a chopped banana, 1 tsp wheatgerm, 1 tbsp plain live yogurt and 1 dsp slivered almonds

Lunch   Cellulite Buster Big Salad (see page 61)
3 fresh apricots or a peach

Dinner   *Starter* – 250ml bowl of watercress or asparagus soup
Main course – Pan-fried salmon, broad beans, peas and broccoli
or – 150g stir-fried tofu cubes with mixed vegetables

Dessert   Mixed fresh fruit salad, including melon, mango and another stoned fruit
or – if it's autumn, apple and blackberries, or at any other season a baked apple with sultanas, served with 1 tbsp half-fat crème fraiche or fromage frais

Savoury   28g cheese, 2 sticks celery, 1 fresh apricots and 6 whole almonds

Exercise   Your choice of buster block
30-minute walk
Full programme of toning exercises

Breakfast   40g (one teacupful) Cellulite Buster Breakfast Muesli (page 82) with a teacupful of skimmed or soya milk
Fruit and yoghurt as Day 1

Lunch   Cellulite Buster Big Salad (see page 61)
An apple

Dinner   *Starter* – 250ml bowl of carrot and coriander soup or a mixed green leaf salad with Parmesan shavings
Main course – Plain foil-roasted cod or salmon fillet, served on mashed potatoes with a Cellulite Buster Small Salad (see page 63) or broad beans or peas
or – Quorn cooked as above and with the same accompaniments

Dessert   A large dish of sliced strawberries topped with 1 tbsp plain live yoghurt or half-fat crème fraiche

Savoury   28g cheese, 2 sticks celery, 2 plums

Exercise   Aerobics video
Full programme of toning exercises

Breakfast 2 eggs, cooked any way you choose with 2 slices of wholegrain toast
Fruit and yoghurt as Day 1

Lunch Cellulite Buster Big Salad (see page 61)
A pear

Dinner *Starter* – Corn on the cob or a mixed salad with toasted pine nuts
Main course – Salade Niçoise (see page 142)
or – as above but without the tuna, and with a sprinkling of Parmesan cheese

Dessert Bowl of strawberries with 2 tbsp half-fat fromage frais
or – a bowl of apple and blackberry with 1 tbsp plain live yoghurt or 1 tbsp half-fat evaporated milk

Savoury 28g Cheddar, Edam or Stilton, 2 sticks celery, 1 peach and a few cherries

Exercise 50-minute power walk
100 bottom squeezes
20 all-fours gluteal and hamstring toner
100 bottom squeezes
20 all-fours gluteal and hamstring toner
20 hip toning lifts to each side
Inner thigh toner

Breakfast   Cellulite Buster Protein Shake (page 147)
2 slices Multigrain toast with sugar-free orange spread

Lunch   Large Waldorf Salad or Cellulite Buster Big Salad (see pages 147, 61)

Dinner   *Starter* – 250ml bowl of vegetable or lentil soup
Main course – Chicken with Peaches (see page 141), served with dark leaf salad including watercress, and a Cellulite Buster Small Salad (see page 63)
or – Pan-fried chicken tossed with pine nuts served with salad as above
or – Avocado salad (use a whole avocado) with Parmesan and walnut oil dressing (page 139)

Dessert   Baked peach with 1 tbsp half-fat fromage frais

Savoury   28g low-fat cream cheese, 2 sticks celery and an orange or a pear

Exercise   Your choice of buster block
30-minute power walk
Full programme of toning exercises

Day off (see page 54)

Breakfast   A bowl of banana slices topped with 1 tbsp plain live yogurt and sprinkled with sunflower and pumpkin seeds
A boiled egg with one slice of toast thinly spread with butter

Lunch   Cottage Cheese and Fruit Salad (see page 147)

Dinner   *Starter* – Large mixed salad, including cherry tomatoes and a chopped hard-boiled egg (optional)
Main course – 3-egg omelette with Cellulite Buster Small Salad (see page 63), small jacket potato or 3 small new potatoes (optional)
or – Smoked Salmon with Prawns and Grapes (see page 135)

Dessert   Large dish sliced strawberries topped with 1 tbsp plain live yoghurt or 1 tbsp half-fat crème fraiche
or – a dish of apple and blackberry with 1 tbsp plain live yoghurt
You can have 2 tbsp of half-fat evaporated milk with both dishes if you like

Savoury   28g low-fat cream cheese with garlic and chives, 2 sticks celery, an apple

Exercise   Swim or run/walk programme
30-minute power walk
5 minutes abdominals
Stretching exercise

Breakfast   40g porridge (made with water), topped with as much skimmed or soya milk as you like, but no sugar
Fruit and yoghurt as Day 1

Lunch   Cellulite Buster Big Salad (see page 61)
1 tbsp plain live yoghurt with 1 tbsp fresh or tinned raspberries (not raspberry yogurt)

Dinner   *Starter* – 250ml bowl of watercress or asparagus soup
Main course – Pan-fried chicken breast with Fruit and Nut Slaw (see page 145)
or – Baby Spinach, Potato and Egg Salad (see page 143)

Dessert   Baked Peach in Sherry (see page 150) with 1 tbsp half-fat crème fraiche

Savoury   28g cheese, 2 sticks celery, 1 apricot and 6 whole almonds

Exercise   Your choice of buster block
30-minute power walk
20 top of thigh lifts on each leg
20 side leg lifts on each leg
20 all-fours gluteal and hamstring toner on each leg
Repeat the leg exercises twice
Stretching exercise

Breakfast 2 slices Apricot and Brazil Nut toast (see page 151) with sugar-free orange spread
Fruit and yoghurt as Day 1

Lunch Cottage Cheese and Fruit Salad (see page 147)

Dinner *Starter* – Corn on the cob or 250ml bowl of vegetable soup
Main course – Tuna fish salad with cold new potatoes
or – a baked potato filled with 1tbsp tuna or cottage cheese served with Cellulite Buster Small Salad (see page 63)

Dessert A bowl of plums with 1tbsp plain live yoghurt or 2 tbsp half-fat evaporated milk

Savoury 28g cheese, 2 sticks celery, 2 plums

Exercise 30-minute power walk
Your choice of buster block
No toning programme today EXCEPT the stretching exercise

Breakfast   40g oats soaked overnight or for at least an hour in a teacupful of skimmed or soya milk topped with a chopped banana, 1 tsp wheatgerm, 1 tbsp plain live yogurt and 1 dsp slivered almonds

Lunch   Cellulite Buster Big Salad (see page 61)
A small bowl of 8 whole almonds and 1 dsp raisins

Dinner   *Starter* – Small Waldorf Salad (see page 147)
Main course – Foil-baked cod in milk with roast potato slices (spray with oil), spinach or broad beans and peas
or – Feta and walnut salad, you can use another cheese if you prefer

Dessert   Raspberries and blueberries mixed, with 1 tbsp half-fat crème fraiche

Savoury   28g Cheddar, Edam or Stilton, 2 sticks celery, and a few cherries

Exercise   60-minute power walk
5 minutes of abdominals

Breakfast Cellulite Buster Protein Shake (see page 147)
2 slices of Multigrain toast with sugar-free orange spread

Lunch If you're not having the cheese course tonight have 42g cheese
with 2 sticks celery, an apple and a pear
or – if you are having the cheese course tonight have a Cellulite
Buster Big Salad (see page 61)
An apple

Dinner *Starter* – Mixed salad with walnuts
Main course – Chicken in Orange Marinade (see page 138), but
oven baked rather than grilled, served with broccoli and
cauliflower and potatoes
or – substitute Quorn for the chicken

Dessert Large dish sliced strawberries and raspberries, topped with
1 tbsp half-fat crème fraiche

Savoury 28g cheese, 2 sticks celery, 1 apricot, 6 whole almonds

Exercise Your choice of buster block
Walk
Full programme of toning exercises

Breakfast	A bowl of banana slices topped with 1 tbsp plain live yogurt and sprinkled with sunflower and pumpkin seeds
	A boiled egg with one slice of toast thinly spread with butter
Lunch	Cellulite Buster Big Salad (see page 61)
	A pear
Dinner	*Starter* – 250ml bowl of carrot and coriander soup or leek and potato soup
	Main course – Pan-fried salmon fillet, with stir-fried courgettes, peppers and asparagus
	or – Avocado salad with pine nuts and Parmesan, served on leafy salad including watercress
Dessert	Mixed berries of your choice with half-fat fromage frais
Savoury	28g cheese, 2 sticks celery, 2 plums
Exercise	100 bottom squeezes
	20 all-fours gluteal and hamstring toner
	100 bottom squeezes
	20 all-fours gluteal and hamstring toner
	Repeat this programme twice more then do
	5 minutes of abdominals
	Stretching exercise

Day off (see page 54)

Breakfast   40g porridge (made with water), topped with as much skimmed or soya milk as you like, but no sugar
A bowl of sliced banana and mixed berries topped with 1 tbsp plain live yogurt

Lunch   Cottage Cheese and Fruit Salad (see page 147)

Dinner   *Starter* – Half a melon filled with raspberries
Main course – Plain roast chicken with 2 roast potatoes and two other vegetables, gravy

Dessert   Fresh plums and apricot slices with 1 tbsp plain live yoghurt
or – Baked or stewed apple with 1 tbsp half-fat crème fraiche

Savoury   28g Brie, 2 sticks celery, 2 fresh apricots

Exercise   Your choice of buster block
30-minute power walk
Hip toning lifts – 20 each side
Side leg lifts – 20 each leg
5 minutes of abdominals

Breakfast   2 eggs cooked any way you choose with 2 slices of wholegrain toast

Fruit and yoghurt as Day 1

Lunch   Large Waldorf Salad (see page 147)

Dinner   *Starter* – Corn on the cob

Main course – Barbecued Salmon with Citrus (see page 135) or alternatively bake in foil, served with a mixed salad and 3 boiled new potatoes

or – Avocado and pine nut salad on a bed of watercress and rocket, with a baked potato if required

Dessert   Strawberry, Banana and Peach Kebab (see page 149), topped with 1 tbsp half-fat crème fraiche

Savoury   28g cheese, 2 sticks celery, 2 fresh apricots

Exercise   Aerobics class or video

45-minute power walk

Full programme of toning exercises

Yoga class or video

The Fast Track

Seven day Fast Track

This diet is for emergencies only. It is for people who need a real kick to get started. It is also a good diet to come back to if your weight loss gets stuck or your motivation needs a kick. I haven't included it in the basic Cellulite Buster Diet because I would prefer that you stick with that. But sometimes we all need a little bit of help, so this is the fast track.

Think of a diet as a journey from London to Edinburgh to go to a party. You've driven non-stop for three hours, you're shattered, and there's still another six hours to go. But at least you're heading in the right direction. If you decide the journey's so long that you're not even going to attempt it, you won't get to Edinburgh and you'll save yourself all this anguish – but you'll also miss the party. So which is it going to be?

Well, you could always fly instead of driving and this seven-day optional phase of the Cellulite Buster Diet is the equivalent of saying 'to hell with it – I just want to get there!' It's perfect if you have a problem getting started, and it means that when you get to Phase One you'll feel you have so much more to eat! But there are a few conditions for fast tracking:

— You should be in good health and not be taking any medication.
— You should be at least 10kg above your ideal weight. You can't burn body fat if you haven't got any, so don't try to diet down from 55 kilos to 50 kilos just because you've got a thing about feeling fat.
— Stay on the fast-track for no longer than seven days.
— Don't eat less than the amounts I've given you, even if you think you can. Your metabolism will only slow down to accommodate the lower calorie intake.

Other rules
— No Day Off
— It is important that you stick with the diet for the FULL SEVEN DAYS.

What to drink

Plain bottled or tap water. Normal tea or herbal or fruit teas and decaffeinated coffee.

EVERY DAY

Breakfast

40g oats, microwaved with water and topped with 1 tbs plain live yoghurt, 1 tsp honey, a pinch of cinnamon. A glass of water.

Or, if you are in a hurry and need to take breakfast with you, soak 40g oats in skimmed or soya milk, with toppings as above. You can take this with you in an air-tight container.

Lunch

2 glasses of plain water.

Stir-fried vegetables with lentils and rice

This can be eaten hot or cold.

Stir-fry any amount of mixed vegetables in 1 tbsp sunflower oil.
Choose the vegetables from:

asparagus spears
courgette slices
red and yellow peppers
carrot batons
broccoli florets
onions
peas
bean sprouts
baby corn

Add 1 tbsp tinned green lentils and heat through. This can be seasoned with fresh herbs and soy sauce. Serve on 3 tbsp boiled rice.

Dinner

Dinner is the same cooked salad as you had for lunch but you should add one of the protein foods below:

— 200g chicken breast
— 150g fillet of salmon
— 150g fillet of cod
— 1 tbsp cashew nuts or whole almonds
— 150g pan-fried tofu cubes

If you would like a cold meal, have a large mixed salad including tomatoes, chicory, beetroot, etc.

You should drink at least 2 glasses of spring or filtered water.

Dessert

Half a melon, filled with you choice of and any amount of fresh raspberries, blueberries, strawberries.

2 glasses water.

Mid-evening

Cup warm milk or cup of tea.

1 plain oatcake.

1 apple.

Cravings, Tricky Situations and Setbacks

CRAVINGS

Cravings aren't a fight between you and food. They're a battle between two halves of your brain, one saying, 'Go on, have it, one won't matter' and the other saying, 'Don't!' Cravings can only be conquered when you've put your brain into restraint mode. Don't fall back on the excuse that you can make up for it tomorrow: tomorrow you must eat as normal.

In my research into cravings I found that if someone was told that, for medical reasons, they absolutely couldn't have something – maybe it would interact badly with prescription medication as, for example, do some anti-depressants with cheese and broad beans – they had no trouble resisting. Not only that, but there was no desire for that particular food, no fight or regret. The decision was removed by the greater power of illness or pain. But when you know you shouldn't eat something because it merely interferes with your weight loss, it becomes a fixation. If it were only a matter of deciding whether you want one biscuit, fine, but when people give in to cravings they eat the whole packet – and as if to make sure the damage is well and truly done, they eat a second packet as well! Cravings do strange things to people.

You resist cravings with willpower. Now this is the most elusive of all the virtues because nobody can have willpower for you, but you do have it or you wouldn't have made the decision to start this diet. Abandon the diets that promise a daily 'treat' of something sweet or sugary or fattening ('just this tiny piece!') because they are like offering an alcoholic just half a glass of wine a day as a treat. If you crave sweet things, you're addicted. If you're addicted, you must remove it from your life completely.

Cravings can't last. They need an attention span. Cravings are worse in the evening because there is less to distract you. Once it gets on your mind you'll hunt down that bit of chocolate cake even if it means going to the ends of the earth. You'll eat it frenziedly, as if you hate it for having got the better of you. But if you lived in a remote part of the world where the only available food were rice and vegetables, you wouldn't crave chocolate. Long for it, maybe. Wish you had some. But there wouldn't be any chocolate and gradually the yearning for it would go.

It's like cigarettes. People crave them terribly when they first stop smoking but they don't still crave them terribly six months later. They don't even think about them after ten years. That's because they aren't having the odd cigarette, that little bit of a reminder of what they're missing. People who lose weight but can't keep it off nearly always had diets that allowed daily treats. This isn't to say that everyone who eats chocolate automatically has a craving or a weight problem: we know that's not so. But fancying a slice of cake is different from craving it so badly that you end up on a binge, and it's that behaviour you have to stop. People who stay slim always followed my strict rule of totally banning sweets, biscuits and chocolate. It helps you not only get slim, but stops you backsliding on your diet.

Impulse food buying

Food and its proximity is the same as a pair of shoes in the shop and a credit card. The thought and the action are just seconds apart. If you had to go home and fetch the cash, chances are you wouldn't buy the shoes; you'd have time to think about it rationally. Thinking time allows sensible thought to overtake the impulse. On perhaps three occasions out of ten people will go back for the shoes, but on the other seven occasions they don't, according to surveys carried out by the Consumers Association. This is why shops adore credit cards!

In the world of insurance salesmen and double glazing, this impulse problem has been taken care of by the introduction of 'cooling-off' periods. Impulsive thoughts allied to convincing sales talk adds up to potential disaster. When someone says to me, 'Why can't I stop eating biscuits all evening?' my answer is, 'Because you have them in the house!'

Cravings will stop if:

You have two meals a day to look forward to, which contain enough carbohydrates. Your body needs carbohydrates, but it needs them in measured doses. Having too few carbohydrates, or too many sugary carbohydrates that raise your blood sugar too quickly, mean your sugar levels are swinging around wildly and your body speaks to you in the only way it knows how – it makes you want more sugar. Cravings are more than fancying food – they are a deep physical need, but this diet will remove cravings.

You never allow biscuits, cakes or sweets into the house. Boredom can lead to a vague feeling of restlessness and fancying something sweet. If you have sweet food in the house, you will eat it, but the sensation will disappear if you have nothing to satisfy your sweet tooth. I recommend having fruit, or a good plate of salad with some grated cheese instead.

Clean your teeth and rinse your mouth after every meal. This is a short-term measure that works extremely well if your need for something sweet is only slight. A really strong taste of mint from brushing your teeth will take away the desire to eat.

TRICKY SITUATIONS

Eating out

'What can I eat when I go out?' is the question on most people's lips. Fortunately, a business lunch is easier to deal with than a social lunch or dinner. Here are the points for and against a business lunch:

For
— You get a choice from a menu.
— You can ask for variations and special considerations.
— There is usually a time limit on the meal – people have to get back to work.
— If there is no time limit, you can excuse yourself citing work pressures.

— There is usually an agenda, so people will be more interested in the talk than the food.
— People drink a lot less at lunches now than they used to – nobody thinks it strange if you stick to water.

Against
— Fancy menus.
— Three courses – you can't have nothing if everyone else is eating.
— Unlike a social lunch, it's not meant to be fun.

Best menu choices

Plain fish – Pan-fried or poached. If the menu has a sauce with the dish, ask for it to be served plain.

Plain vegetables – Ask for them to be served plain, without butter or glaze.

Chicken – Roasted, grilled or poached or chicken tikka or tandoori. No sauce. The difference between chicken masala and chicken tikka is more than 400 calories per portion.

Scallops and mussels

Plain lamb fillet – medallions or roast. Avoid curried or casseroled lamb – it can have a lot of fattening ingredients in the sauce.

Beef – Steak is best, plain grilled. Avoid bourguignon, casseroles or curries which are often sealed in oil before cooking, and have additions like onions which are usually softened in butter or oil before being added.

Avoid
Any kind of risotto – even vegetarian ones have a ton of butter in them.

Desserts and puddings

— Fresh fruit, fruit salads, etc. If there is nothing but fruit-topped flans and pies you must eat only the fruit and leave the pastry. If anyone asks (which they shouldn't), say, 'I'm not mad about pastry.' Whatever you do, don't say you're watching your waistline, counting calories or any of the other boring things that people say. You'll never hear the end of it.

— Cheese and celery. This is not a strange choice – switching to cheese from the traditional sweet course might have more calories and fat, but it will stop you backsliding into the old world of sweet things which fuels that old sweet tooth. Cheese often comes with grapes, so pick at these – it will look like you're joining in, being sociable and enjoying yourself.

— If there is nothing suitable, take another look at the starter menu. It might have something like melon or grapefruit, so ask for that instead. Nobody will care.

Three courses

It isn't good manners to sit and eat nothing when others choose three or more courses. Don't see this as the end of your diet. You might not want a starter, but you'll be used to the simple list of starters I've given you, and these are all low-calorie and nutritious. Choose shellfish, fruit or clear soup.

Accompaniments

'Does it come with anything?' you should ask when you survey a devilishly complicated item on a menu. Sometimes, vegetables are your only salvation from an amalgamation of foods piled into a tower, which is the fashionable way to serve meals these days. You can't possibly know how each element was cooked, although the good thing is that these meals tend to be tiny. It is almost impossible to get anything simple in the type of restaurants that have a couple of stars attached to them, so save on the accompaniments – don't have any.

If it has to go on a separate plate, you don't need it

Your side plate is redundant. If it is the sort of restaurant that gives you bread without a plate, this isn't an excuse to cheat! Bread is out. Nibbles are out. Appetisers or anything else masquerading as a stop-gap are out. Have a drink before your first course but have nothing else. After all, you're about to eat a meal. You're hardly going to collapse from hunger.

Alcohol

I wouldn't drink at lunch. This has nothing to do with calories, but we all know that alcohol weakens resolve. You promise yourself 'just one' but by the time the bottle comes round again you're more relaxed, mellow and likely to shrug your shoulders and say you'll diet tomorrow. Tomorrow comes, and you decide to just have one more day before you start again. It's not an inevitable scenario, but it happens. Most of my clients say they fell off the wagon food-wise when they'd had too much to drink. Phrases like 'what's life about?' and 'you only live once' came to mind. Next day they realized what life was about: being plastered wasn't all it was cracked up to be.

While you're slimming, stay off the booze. Take it in four-week spells, and every time you're on a 'diet month', put your mind into 'method mode'. That means you're a non-drinker!

The social lunch or dinner

These are meals in people's houses and I'm afraid you've got to get through them the best way you can. The days of four different puddings and a choice of starters is long gone. Nowadays you're likely to get nibbles with the first drink, a set starter, main course, pudding, cheese and chocolates. All with accompanying wines. It depends on the company you keep, but if you're into serious country-house dining or big-time, best-manners, work-related dinners, people will arrive up to an hour late and think nothing of it. If you've been one of the first to arrive, you'll be waiting for your meal for ages, and be desperate to lay into the nuts and cheese straws. Eat before you go!

This can be something like a salad, your starter salad, for example, or some fruit. You might just want to wait and be hungry, and that won't hurt either. But do beware of this trap because an extra 600–800 calories can slip down your throat before you even get going on the actual meal. Probably best to turn up late yourself.

In the country you'll probably get standard warming fare like crumbles and a good roast and the only way round this is to eat small portions and have a second helping of vegetables. Personally, I always take the view that I'm not going to eat anything I don't want to eat, and eating until my skirt is straining isn't a compliment to my hostess. Enjoying the meal is enough in itself, and you can't enjoy it any more because you've been a glutton. A meal is only a strain on your system if you allow it to be, so eat the meat and vegetables, go easy on gravy, stuffings, sausages (if it's a Christmas do) and all the extras, and, if you can, pick around the crumble and eat the fruit. It's very important that you don't eat the crumble topping or Yorkshire puddings or stuffing while you're cellulite busting. It's not a good idea to keep allowing yourself a lapse or just one pudding, even if it's your day off. It depends on the lapse, but one leads to another, so get to know yourself. Go easy, you're getting rid of your cellulite and losing weight!

In towns, by the way, life can be easier. People tend to ring ahead of time and explain that they can't eat this or that, or have an unusual intolerance, and nobody seems to think anything of it.

My advice is don't invent an intolerance. While other people will remember it, you'll forget and they'll pounce on you the next time you pick up a piece of bread (or whatever it was you said you couldn't eat). Here are some tried-and-tested rules for getting through a meal out, especially useful when you're rightly determined not to let your diet slip!

— Say you're driving – nobody presses alcohol on someone who's driving.
— Take everything that's offered. The minute you decline something it draws attention to the fact and someone might pipe up, 'Not on a diet, are you?' (This isn't good manners, but there's no accounting for the other guests your hosts have invited, and believe me, once someone looks as if she's on a diet, there's nowhere to hide. It happens particularly when you're already slim: if you're overweight you can relax because everyone's too embarrassed to mention it.)
— You can't refuse a beef bourguignon at a private dinner, so in case your hostess happens to have fried everything off in a litre of butter and added double cream, restrict yourself to a moderate portion. If you're really desperate that your diet could be sabotaged, and you know yourself better than I do, you could corner your hostess and mutter something about cholesterol, but I wouldn't bother. She'll be too hassled to care, or if she does, she'll feel guilt-ridden for not providing an alternative. Eat up and shut up is the best policy.
— The way to play this is to take all the vegetables, bread or sauce with enthusiasm, fiddle around with it and leave whatever you don't want. In my experience, people notice that your plate was

full and you were eating – they never notice how much you left. A half-full plate from the outset looks terrible, and is more of a slap in the face for your hostess.

— Drink masses of water. It takes time and it fills you up.
— Eat all the vegetables, and by all means have seconds.
— Have your day off and allow a bit of everything.

Shift work

Shift work isn't the minefield you think it is. The rule is the same for everyone; eat a main meal when you wake and eat a main meal at the end of your work, before you relax. If you come home and go straight to bed, you should eat a couple of hours before you sleep. Always have a light meal in the middle of your working shift. Whatever happens, you mustn't allow the work to get in the way of your health, which is a trend I notice from my mailbag. Carry a meal with you. This is the sort of thing you can plan:

— On your days off work, make your salads and cereals, and buy enough fruit for the week. Make sure you have some snap-shut containers to take salads and previously stir-fried vegetables and bits to work.
— Remember to cook an extra piece of fish or chicken with every main meal. If you can't do that, use tinned tuna fish or slice half an avocado and add it to your Cellulite Buster Big Salad. This is a nutritious meal to take to work with you.
— When you come home, or if you need a savoury breakfast, microwave a potato and have it with your Cellulite Buster Small Salad.
— Never go to bed on an empty stomach. If you're too tired to eat, have your breakfast meal of oats with fruit, but don't have bread before bed – it's too indigestible.

Fitting in with the family

It isn't always convenient to cook separate meals for the family, and what you want most of all is to cook just one meal. This leads to a dilemma, and a dilemma that causes a lot of weight problems. Either the family is going to eat your fish and salads, to which the answer is 'I don't think so!' or you are going to have something separate. This isn't a major problem, so let's plan:

— You only have six meals a week to worry about – nobody worries about what they're going to eat for breakfast

— A couple of those meals will be things that everyone likes – probably chicken. Try omelettes one day too. Make yours with salad, potatoes can be shared by everyone, and add whatever they like.

— You now only have three or four meals that might be different if they don't like fish. It's not a big deal, so for families I usually recommend doing the roast or poached fish option. There's nothing easier than putting a dish in the oven with a piece of fish in it, or even microwaving it. Potatoes are pretty universal, and most children love peas and sweetcorn.

— Don't forget that feeding your children this sort of diet is only going to be good for them so don't let them get away with battered or bread-crumbed meals!

SETBACKS

The 'plateau'

Well, you always said that diets don't work. It's easy to trot that out when you've got friends round and your weight's gone up again. Some people feel an enormous antagonism towards dieting, and hate themselves for having to go on one. They say that diets don't work when in fact what they mean is that they couldn't find a diet they could live with. Or stick to.

But what is a diet, for heaven's sake? A diet is just a mode of eating, just as a cat's diet is meat and a sheep's diet is grass. Some diets are aimed at less energy and these are slimming diets. So why don't they work?

They do. Let me give you an analogy: an elite athlete trains and competes in a particular way and keeps getting injured. One day he has a sudden severe injury and he is taken to hospital for a major operation. After six months' recuperation, he is pronounced fit enough to start training again, he trains the same way and lo and behold, he is soon back writhing on the ground in agony. Does this mean the operation was a failure?

Of course not. He's simply gone back to doing whatever caused the injury in the first place. If you go on doing the same thing, the same thing will happen. It doesn't mean the athlete cannot play his sport again, but he must do it differently – on different surfaces with different shoes, perhaps. In extreme cases people have even been known to have their running style analysed by computer to see if they have problems with posture or gait, and this has proved remarkably successful in correcting problems and bringing about amazing success. What this story tells us is that if something hasn't worked for you in the past, it doesn't mean that it was useless and it doesn't mean you were useless. It means that you went back to whatever caused the problems before you started the diet. Analysing your problems and trying different diets is a good idea. Diets do work, but you have to live with them, and you will get to this later on when I explain about going into Phase Two of the plan – coasting. You won't be on a diet, you will 'have' a diet.

The plateau is the stage at which your weight loss has stalled. It happens to everybody. When I tell people that their weight will start to fall again, they never believe me. Your body is gradually re-adjusting to your lower weight. You metabolic rate is set by the amount of muscle (lean tissue) in your body, and your size. The smaller you are, the less energy you need. The plateau is a sign that you are lighter, so be glad of it. Take these steps:

— If you are on Phase Two, go back to Phase One for two weeks. If you're desperate, like a date's coming or you won't fit into your wedding dress, do seven days on the fast track.

— Increase your AEROBIC exercise by 30 minutes a day or change your toning exercise for aerobic exercise, if you can't spare an extra 30 minutes.

— Drink more water – this will flush out excess fluids.

— Check that you don't have a period coming – this can add over 2 kilos to your weight.

— Cut out the evening potatoes for one week. This is not the best measure, as you shouldn't cut back too much on calories, but you might have been eating more than you thought.

— Finally, don't think that just because you can't see weight loss, it isn't happening. You can't see your hair growing either!

The art of living goes hand-in-hand with the art of a good diet. A good diet is all about eating properly. You need to spend time on it and not hold back from spending money on it, especially never spending more on clothes than you would on good food. If you follow these guidelines, you will have the most fabulous body you ever dreamed of.

Your questions answered

You use a lot of butter in your recipes, especially for pan-frying. I'm worried about the fat content of the diet – it can't be right, surely?

I know what you mean. There's a difference between a high-fat diet and meals which have a lot of fat in them, and I'll explain. Pan-frying in a little butter is fine. Most of it is still in the pan when you take out the chicken or fish, and the small amount that sears the outside of the food is hardly going to kill you. Remember that butter is a natural, wholesome ingredient – it only matters when you're eating it at every meal, every day, for months and years on end.

Having butter or cheese at the odd meal still keeps your diet lower in total fat than one with, say daily biscuits and cake. Do bear that in mind.

I work in a hotel on shifts and when I'm on earlies I have to eat breakfast there. It's whatever they can be bothered to provide and usually consists of white toast, cornflakes and eggs. What can I have?

Well, you're not on every day, so that's something. Perhaps you could take your own packet of muesli and keep it tucked away on a shelf or in your locker? It doesn't matter if you can only have full-fat milk – once a day won't hurt. Take some fruit slices in a snap-shut container as well. I find that people who really want to manage, manage very well. It would be the same if you were on a special diet for medical reasons, so treat it like that. It's a shame to have to spend your own money on a meal that should be free, but it's better than eating what they provide, and it won't cost much.

I hate vegetables! I really, really can't stand the smell or taste of any of them, and my diet is usually chicken, potatoes, fruit, rice and pasta. I have terrible cellulite though and I'm desperate to do something. What else can I eat?

Unfortunately, the Cellulite Buster Diet has lots of vegetables because of their amazing properties. They help your body's natural detox processes and have lots of precious fibre. This is all part of the treatment for cellulite.

I'm sure there are ways that you could manage to eat vegetables, perhaps in a vegetable curry or soup? But I can't compromise on something that is essential – it's like leaving something out in a cake recipe and expecting it to turn out perfect. If you can't eat vegetables there isn't a substitute I'm afraid, and this diet won't really be suitable for you.

I'm impressed by the fact that I don't have to go to a gym. I have quite a lot of spare time as I'm unemployed – can I do more exercise than you've recommended?

Yes you can. As long as you don't do a lot of the same thing, it's another way of fast tracking yourself. Don't add extra toning or weight exercises – power walking and jogging or swimming are good ideas. If you overdo it, you could end up flat on your back with overuse injury, so make a total of no more than 1 ½ hours a day, plus your usual general activity.

I've been doing the diet for the thirty days and a further five weeks, and my willpower is waning – especially round my time of the month. Now I'm not so strict with myself it seems I've let myself go and can't get back. What should I do?

Go back and do seven days fast track, and seven days of Phase One. Then re-try Phase Two. If you have a permanent problem with willpower, I've known great success from people who 'layer' their phases in a four-week cycle, like this:

— 2 weeks of Phase Two before your period
— 1 week Phase One during your period
— 1 week fast track after your period

I'm interested in the presentation side. My legs have got nice and slim but my skin is still blotchy and uneven. I don't feel I can go out without tights.

I've always found leg make-up an indispensable item in my beauty bag. Found in high street chemists, it's usually called 'Stocking Cream' or something similar. You need to rub a blob of it between your palms before you apply it to moisturized legs, as a little goes a very long way. Waterproof and smudge proof, you could even leave it on while you sleep and have hardly any smears on the sheets. (Depends what kind of a night you have!) It makes legs look smooth and blemish free, and nobody will know you're wearing leg make-up.

In previous books, you've said that you've kept the same weight through managing total calories and keeping carbohydrates low. In this diet you've recommended bread for breakfast and potatoes in the evening. Cereals are also high carbohydrate and there's all that fruit! I'm not sure what to believe now.

First of all, it's horses for courses. Why isn't there one general-purpose contraceptive pill when all we want to do is prevent pregnancies? We're all different and whatever pill you get has the same effect, and a diet is no different. So do be open to new ways.

You rightly point out that this diet has bread and potatoes plus other carbohydrate food. But that doesn't make it high in carbohydrates. A typical day, with bread for breakfast, corn on the cob as a starter and a portion of potatoes, plus plenty of fruit and vegetables, would come to about 166g carbohydrate, broken down like this:

2 slices bread – 32g
banana – 23g
Cellulite Buster Big Salad – 8g
apple – 11g
corn on the cob – 14.5g
chicken and vegetable stir-fry – 7.3g
portion potatoes – 30g
bowl plums or cherries – 12g
yoghurt – 10g
TOTAL – 147.8g

This is still below the recommended daily average for an active woman which is 180–250g, and the reason for this is that sugar is the item with the highest carbohydrate punch of all – two sweet pancakes give you 77g carbohydrate and one Danish pastry packs a stunning 56.4g carbohydrate, all for a snack!

Do remember that even a low-carbohydrate diet can make you gain weight if you eat too much fat, and vice versa. It's the diet as a whole that causes the problems.

My legs are unbelievably awful. From a tiny waist I balloon to huge tree trunks. I've been like this all my life, with thick knees and ankles. I've managed by wearing trousers all the time, but I know those legs are lurking underneath and it make me shy of stripping off. Surely this plan can't work for me?

Yes it can. The problem with something that you've had for as long as you can remember is that you've accepted it as part of your life and it's become a problem that's part of you. You've always worn trousers. Generally speaking, people don't even begin a diet and exercise plan when all they can remember is that their legs were fat.

You weren't born with fat and lumpy muscles. It doesn't matter why you're like this, but fat can be removed. Muscles can be toned and stretched. You just haven't had a really good go at it.

This might take you longer than thirty days, but the journey is a series of stages, so you don't suddenly go from 'awful' to 'gorgeous' without anything in between. People forget that they're improving all the time. The most important exercise for you will be walking and running plus sustained stretching, so do my walk/run programme daily.

About stretching. Stretching hurts. Most people stop the minute it hurts and never get any better. Persevere with it because it doesn't hurt for more than half a minute.

I want to do the fast track more often – say one week a month. Isn't this too few calories?

There's a lot of debate about calories and so-called crash diets. I am utterly convinced by research in America that proves low-calorie diets actually slow down the ageing process, and being a little on the thin side – as long as it is what I call 'healthy-thin' – is the recipe for a healthy long life. As far as your legs and bottom are concerned, low-calorie in particular and less food generally is the way to go. People get very anxious about not having enough to eat, and I understand that. Eating is a pleasurable and sociable thing to do. But you can still enjoy pleasant sociable meals without packing in enough calories for an army. I think we have to accept these days that we just don't have the same energy needs as we once did (and I include myself in that), whether it's due to getting older generally or from being lazier by having cars and central heating, the evidence is there on your lower half. There's no shortcut – you've got to eat less. Yes, it's fine to do the fast track once a month as long as you don't extend it to a second week – keep to the standard coasting plan for the rest of the time or the general Cellulite Buster Diet if you still need to lose weight steadily.

I've got five children, including twins, all under six years of age. I can't possibly find time for a special exercise plan. How can I fit it in?
You can't. There comes a time when you have to admit that you can't be all things to all people, and the drawbacks of being so busy are outweighed by the benefits – you have five healthy children!

Sometimes you have to accept that you've swapped one set of good things for another. Nobody who has had a baby or two has the same body that she had before the babies – how could she? You can find a short cut to lovely legs through diet and this will help you to feel more energetic and to look healthy. If you really can't find time for exercise though – and you clearly can't – you might find the presentation section useful for making your cellulite appear less of a problem.

I used to be incredibly slim. Now I've let things slide and have gained 12 kilos, all on my legs and bum. I can't seem to motivate myself to be strict any more. What's wrong with me?
It's easy to let your desires drift. If something seems like hard work, then why do it today any more than tomorrow? Or next week? People feel this way about a variety of tasks, especially paying bills or phoning people. It's the easiest thing in the world to pick up a phone or write that cheque, but sometimes you practically have to put a gun to your head to galvanize yourself into any kind of action. I am sure this rings a bell with you, because we all do it about something in our lives. On other occasions you're strong and positive. Strength of purpose is important when it comes to willpower, because if there is no real purpose beyond 'getting rid of cellulite' or 'losing weight' you have no driving force. If you had to do it before someone would give you a job, your purpose would be there.

Your compelling reason must be your image of yourself. You also have to give yourself a timescale. Don't let this drift and don't let weakness of mind take over. Tomorrow won't do. Get that mental image of your great body firmly in your mind and look forward to it becoming reality. Looking back to when things went wrong is your downfall.

What is cellulite and how can I hope to have thinner thighs? – they're in the family!

Lots of women have excess fat on their legs and bottoms without having cellulite. Others have cellulite despite being thin. For all the theories that abound, nobody has come up with an explanation and to be honest – do we really care? We want to get rid of it as quickly as possible, and you shouldn't pay any attention to the genetic theory. I honestly don't think that fat is the whole story, and I lay the blame at the door of bad diet. People will say sportswomen have no cellulite, but I think that's because they eat properly. You can't run a marathon or swim the Channel on a packet of crisps and a Mars bar. Exercise is vitally important because it helps get rid of fluid and waste build-up. Anybody who's been ill for a time or bedridden will tell you that however much fruit and vegetables they eat, they still get constipated. Movement matters.

It's not an accident that the place we get cellulite just happens to be the place that takes two-thirds of our weight for hours on end every day when we sit on it! And if you know someone who never moves a muscle, eats like a horse and drinks like a fish and has fabulously cellulite-free legs, you can be assured of one thing – it's on its way.

Some women tend to lay down fat stores on their hips, thighs and buttocks. Others store fat on their stomachs and have thin legs. Some people are fat all over. Whether you're a pear or an apple – or neither – does tend to run in families, but you're not doomed. Genetics are only a tendency, not an inevitability. I can absolutely promise that if you decide you are going to get rid of your cellulite, you will.

Exercise

Most people would rather eat a bit less than exercise. Trouble is, losing all the fat in the world won't make your legs look good. It might not even make your cellulite disappear. Fat always hangs on to the bitter end in the places that get the least movement – and that means your bottom. Exercising your body is not an option, in the same way that you can't just decide you never want to take your dog for a walk. It has to be done. So grin and bear it, and remember that you're going to end up the winner.

Fat and muscle are totally different. Burning fat will make you slimmer and healthier, toned muscles will make you look firm. Put together, they're a magic combination for a great-looking body that will attract attention for years and years. After all, if you look good at twenty, nobody thinks it's anything special: looking just as good at forty really gets you noticed!

This plan is quite challenging. For thirty days you need to schedule in at least an hour and fifteen minutes of special exercise every day, but it's more than worth it. The results you get depend on the amount of effort you put in, and stop–starting a programme will get you nowhere. So go for it! The only thing you'll be losing is your cellulite and those extra inches.

What is toning?

Muscles are attached to tendons or bones, and they're with you from birth. You can't lose them or get rid of them through lack of use. They don't suffer long-term after a caesarean delivery or other operation (bang goes that old excuse then!). In really bad circumstances, say for example, where someone has been bedridden for years the muscles would be very thin and weak but they'd still be there. Their potential to be firm and healthy and strong again would be there too. However much you think you've let yourself go, you can always climb back. When somebody says,

'I'm just a hopeless case, a lost cause' my answer's always, 'There's no such thing.'

A muscle is a series of long fibres. When you exercise a muscle (think of a biceps curl holding a weight) the muscle is contracted and relaxed, contracted and relaxed. As you pump away, the muscle works against the weight and the fibres begin to burn as they work harder. The blood flow increases and you get hot. This is toning. It happens during normal activities too: washing the car, lifting the bucket, doing big circular movements with your arms all involve contracting and relaxing muscles. Heat is generated, you sweat and more calories are brought in as fuel. You can never achieve the same visual result by calorie control alone, because all that does is give you fewer calories while leaving your muscles to stagnate. Diet and exercise attacks from both ends, so you're limiting calories coming in and burning them faster on the way out. It's the best and fastest way to lose weight, and the brilliant thing is that you don't even have to go near a gym.

The more repetitious you make the exercise, the better. The heavier the weight, the more tired your fibres will become. In the couple of days, until you exercise again, the fibres will start to develop because the strain they're under causes them to need more power. You're not aware of this. They don't change while you're exercising, they develop while you're resting. While you are happily watching TV or sleeping, your muscles are recruiting more staff – getting reinforcements if you like. This is how bodybuilders get so incredibly bulky, by using increasingly heavier weights and so forcing muscles to change size. It's amazing what muscles are capable of. Don't get worried that you're going to end up with huge bulging legs, because you won't. With light, repetitious exercise, using nothing heavier than your own bodyweight, your muscles will gradually get stronger, leaner, longer and firmer – not bigger.

Put next to the capabilities of fat, which are nil, you can see how muscles can really work for you. Washing a car isn't exactly the heavy workload I'm making it sound, but the principle's the same. Washing a car demands back-up from all the muscles in your body. Bending, stretching, reaching – they perform a variety of movements, and the payoff comes in that precious recovery time when you need to re-fuel. Remember re-fuelling?

I have explained why you should eat a good meal in the evening. If you've spent a day doing a variety of toning movements like going up and down stairs, carrying shopping and of course doing specific exercise like running, your muscles will be on overtime while you're resting. That evening meal is vital. It won't turn to fat, I promise. If you're active, you can eat – you must eat!

Boosting circulation

General activity also stops your circulation getting sluggish. People like me tend to go on about doing things 'the old way' like getting up to change TV channels rather than using the remote, or walking to the postbox instead of dropping the mail off as you drive by, but these activities are worth a thousand times more to you than an hour a day in the gym. Your heart needs to work faster. Your blood must have more oxygen. A sluggish circulation makes you feel tired because those hardly there breaths scarcely fill a corner of your lungs with oxygen. When you get tired you don't want to exercise, so you lie on the sofa or go to bed, starting the whole cycle that led to the cellulite. If you don't use those muscles, they've got nothing to do. When fat starts to settle, it seeks out the quiet corners where it won't be disturbed.

Fat isn't attached to anything. It sits either in lumps, or in streaks between the bundles of fibres in your muscles. Fat isn't responsible for movement. So basically, fat must be lost and muscles must be used. Do both, and you're on the way to a great-looking body!

How exercise helps with cellulite

As I've said, fat loves little places where it can go unrecognized. Parts of your body that get the most movement get the least fat. You don't gain 5 kilos on your forearms. Your legs might not be your favourite bits, but nobody spreads by 12 centimetres on their ankles or calves. Hands are always doing something. Legs are being crossed and uncrossed, moving car pedals, feet shifting constantly. You only have to think about your entire mid-section from just above your waist to just above your knees and you'll know that this bit of you gets the least movement. Not only do you put a massive 70 per cent of your whole bodyweight on your backside (and lower spine – hence lower back pain) every time you sit down, but you leave it there. Through hours of TV, nights in the pub, through studying and surfing the net. While those hands and arms are busy, your midsection does nothing and the fat settles.

To get great legs therefore, you've got to move them. Now, you're probably thinking, 'But I do! I go to the gym for an hour five times a week – I always take the stairs. I'm on the go all day with my two-year-old!' Well, sorry, but that's not quite what I had in mind!

An hour in the gym, by anyone's standards, is great. But it depends what you do there. In the thirty-day Cellulite Buster Diet, I've given you some different exercise programmes to choose from, which vary according to your starting point. Even if you're an experienced exerciser, you might need to change things around a bit. So how do you exercise? I get asked this a lot by puzzled and frustrated women who understandably need a bit more information than 'do more exercise'. I agree that you want it set out for you, unambiguously.

Vary it

Wandering round the gym, programme card in hand, doing the same old exercises which you simply adapt by doing them a bit longer, is doomed to failure. It will keep you fit, but it won't allow you to progress. It could also do you harm. Your muscles work in pairs, and if you don't work opposing pairs equally you could end up with over-use injuries and pain from one strong muscle group pulling you out of alignment. Do something different each day, but write down a programme to suit your lifestyle, pin it up and then do it. The flip side of this is that you shouldn't vary the routine too much within that activity. It's important not to lift weights every day, but when you do lift weights, don't do a minute of one muscle group, a minute of another and so on, just to try and get some variety going. It's better than not doing it, but you'll get better results by concentrating that session on maybe three or four muscle groups only. This is how you see results.

Consistency

Moving on from what I've just said, you might give up when you don't see results. Going all-out on those few muscle groups is brilliant, but if you miss next week's session, can only manage half a session the week after and so on, you won't have any results and you won't look different. This is such a shame, because your efforts will have been pretty pointless. I know I said that doing some exercise is better than not doing it, but that only applies when you're talking about a walk in the fresh air when you're feeling stale, or a bike ride to keep your hips from getting stiff. If your aim is to lose cellulite and tone up properly, you have to be consistent, start a programme and stay with it for several months. Saying you can't see an instant difference to your shape is like saying you've given up on your hair because you want it to grow 10 centimetres and after a month you can't notice a thing. Not seeing a difference is not the same thing as there not being a difference. That's where your warts-and-all photograph comes in of course, because people never notice the changes in themselves. Then you meet someone you haven't seen for six months and they say, 'Goodness, you've lost weight!'

You'll never hear those golden compliments if you give up.

Consistency means keeping going in spite of temptations to stop. In spite of it being inconvenient. In spite of your cash running out. There's always something you can do. When I go and stay in a hotel in some God-awful town or city and I've got the whole evening stretching out before me, I go for a walk. It might be round roads of boring houses, but there's always something fascinating, even if it's no more than how dreadful they look, or their pretty front gardens or the notices you can read on community boards. I've spent many hours trekking round estates or playing fields. In the hotel room itself, I've done press-ups alternated with sit-ups. Press-ups don't need any equipment but they keep your chest toned. All this is keeping up the consistency of your exercise. Saying, 'Oh, I had to go away on business, so the exercise got kicked into touch for a week,' is a cop-out. However busy you are or however hectic the schedule, whether you're abroad or at home, there's always a quiet moment before dinner or before you go to bed or before breakfast when you can go for a walk, do a few leg lifts or a bit of running on the spot. Even if you're the president of a huge company, you're not president twenty-four hours a day. You're a woman like the rest of us and you get cellulite and flabby legs however much money you've got. Consistency is one of the most important aspects of looking after your body. Your legs don't appreciate being busy one day and idle for the next three. Start your exercise plan with this book, and make it your lifelong commitment to yourself.

It's worth pointing out here that playing games with children is a good way to exercise legs and bottoms. I mean a really good way! Netball, hopscotch, skipping and so on are all toning and stretching exercises which get right to the heart of cellulite country and give it a good blasting. Alternatively, I've just come back from a weekend of walking a coastal path which was incredibly rocky, and fit though I am, my whole lower body is stiff and nicely achy – it must have really put my muscles through their paces. Do take every opportunity to climb, run or simply walk as much as you can.

Your Plan

Follow this plan for your first thirty days.

Aerobic exercise

Aerobic exercise brings life to your lifeless bits. It brings blood to your muscles and sets those fibres in motion. As your circulation pumps round your veins and your muscles move with fast, repetitive movements, more oxygen comes into your body to help cells renew. Cellulite doesn't stand a chance. Current advice is for three sessions of aerobic exercise every week, but I don't think this is nearly enough, especially if you have a sedentary lifestyle. Keep the area moving. Get up and down from your chair, walk as much as you can. At the very least you must do what I'll call your buster block of exercise every day (see opposite) – which is thirty minutes of real heart-stopping stuff. PLEASE don't say you can't find time for thirty minutes – if you do everything else a bit more quickly, be more efficient about reading the newspaper or magazines or simply give up the time you call yours for relaxing, you'll find that amount of time easily.

You don't even have to leave the house. Friends of mine who are airline stewardesses, and who share a house, find they get home at all hours, and therefore can't go to the gym or for a walk because it could be the middle of the night. Instead, they change into leggings and trainers and alternate running up and down the stairs with press-ups, lunges and squats. It's a good programme to get into, so while one is doing twenty stair runs, the other is doing the other stuff, and so on. It works well, and the best thing, they tell me, is that they've done something for themselves, and it feels good. It can't be coincidence that they happen to be absolutely gorgeous too!

Buster blocks

A buster block is your daily thirty-minute session of heart-pumping exercise. You'll be doing this six days a week for thirty days, then you can relax down to five days, then three days on and one day off continuously.

Here are some ideas for buster blocks:

— *Walk/run* – 100 paces of each, for thirty minutes (see page 120–1).

— *Swimming* – Alternate ten lengths with aerobic moves for the backs of the legs, holding the edge of the pool. Straight alternating leg lifts, done slowly, are really effective. Do twenty with each leg, then do ten lengths again.

— *Fast cycling* – It is better to cycle with little resistance (i.e. not up hills) so you don't build up massive muscles. If you're on a stationary bike, do five minutes to warm up, five minutes slightly faster, then go for it incredibly fast for fifteen minutes before slackening off the pace and cooling down for the last five minutes.

— *Brisk uphill walking* – You can't walk uphill for ever, so make the first five minutes a normal walk, then go uphill for at least fifteen minutes. Coming back down (if you're on a real slope not a treadmill) can be tricky for your back, so take care.

— *Aerobics video tape* – My *Get Back Into Your Jeans* workout tape has twenty minutes of aerobics with plenty of arm movements. You finish with lots of leg work for that cellulite too.

— *Stair running* – It's hard to do thirty minutes of stair running, so I suggest you combine it with something else. For example, go for a run or a brisk walk (I mean brisk – you should be walking at a rate of four miles an hour which you can test by walking a mile out and a mile back, in thirty minutes). Then run/walk up and down a flight of stairs twenty times, do some leg lifts, and repeat the sequence for fifteen minutes. Tough, but at least it doesn't cost anything, and you'll have a handy armchair to collapse into when it's all over! This should take about forty-five minutes.

You don't have to do all of these activities in one week, but don't stick with only one of them either. Try three different activities each week – it helps to keep your body in perfect balance if some muscles get a rest while others are put through their paces.

On top of this, you should have a thirty-minute walk every day. I also suggest you do the complete programme of toning exercises (see toning below) on some days, and on others concentrate on only a couple of the exercises. This is quite a challenging programme, but it is vital that you see these thirty days as the real 'busting' part of the plan. Walk during your lunch break. Go round the block a few times and have lunch when you get back. Get up earlier than usual for a thirty-minute trot down the road or to buy the paper. Have a walk before you eat in the evenings. I don't know your personal circumstances, but a friend of mine got into walking when she started going to the postbox with the day's mail every night before bed. It was only up the road and took ten minutes there and back. Then one night the moon looked fantastic, so she decided to make the most of it and walk a bit further. She started going as far as her friend's house, then after a month she was going to the church; before long she wouldn't go to bed until she's walked right round the village. It took her twenty-five minutes, but those minutes added up to just under three hours walking a week. She lost 4.5 kilos in ten months without doing anything else.

If you've got heavy responsibilities at home, do consider a treadmill if you've got the space. I'm normally dead against any kind of equipment, but another friend of mine is completely tied to the house with an elderly mother, and her daily treadmill walk while watching the news has been a lifesaver, keeping her cellulite- and flab-free. I also have a treadmill for use in really bad weather, and I can't recommend it highly enough – as long as it's just for emergencies.

How to walk

No, it's not insulting your intelligence to tell you how to walk! Walking, which is no more than a trudge, doesn't get to the parts you need to target for beautiful smooth legs and bottom. Walking primarily works the hip muscles, the gluteus medius muscles which are what you rest your fists on when you put your hands on your hips in indignation. These muscles stop you falling over to the side like a rag doll, and they work together with your outer thigh muscles. They're important, but they won't dent your cellulite.

To use your hamstrings and gluteus maximus, you must do the following:

— Walk uphill with massive strides. Do it for no less than twenty minutes once you get fit, starting with ten minutes if you're overweight or are new to it.

— Walk up and down stairs, going two at a time when you can. Try walking up and down twice, running once, repeat twice more, then progress to walking twice and running twice, adding an extra running set each time until you can run up and down eight times.

— Step on and off a step or bottom stair. This tones your thigh muscles particularly, but each step up, especially if you step two at a time, uses the buttocks really well. Change leading leg after every twelve steps.

Running

Any form of jogging or running is brilliant aerobic exercise, and will get your circulation going perfectly. I suggest you work up to this plan, which is hard:

— walk 100 paces, run 20 paces
— walk 100 paces run 50 paces
— walk 100 paces, run 100 paces
— repeat 3 more times
— walk 50 paces, run 150 paces
— walk 50 paces, run 200 paces
— run flat-out for five minutes
— walk for ten minutes
— stop and stretch

Swimming

If you haven't any swimming facilities nearby, don't worry, but swimming is fabulous for legs and cellulite. The breaststroke is brilliant and the crawl is absolutely fantastic for the buttocks, with those little flipping movements with straight legs.

If you don't swim, you can still hold onto the side of the pool, let your legs go straight out behind you and do leg movements, as in aqua aerobics. You need to keep going for twenty to thirty minutes to make it work.

Aerobics video

My video *Get Back Into Your Jeans* is still the best-loved aerobics video for a whole generation of long-limbed beauties who I taught during the 1990s. Fast-paced but not complicated, it has twenty minutes of aerobics followed by twenty-five minutes of solid toning. It is still available (see page 154 or log on to HYPERLINK "http://www.monicagrenfell.co.uk" to order). Alternatively, if you're starting from scratch you'll love my *Top To Toe* video, which has an easy segment for total beginners and a second segment which is a bit more challenging. Both target your cellulite with a vengeance!

Stretching

When your muscles are hot, it's time to stretch them. It's like stretching chewing-gum that's been in your mouth for ages – it goes into a long thin string. Try to stretch a piece that's just out of the packet and it just snaps in two. That's how it is with muscles. Don't let this time go to waste, because those precious fifteen minutes after you've worked out are the key to really sensational, long and lean limbs.

Toning

You need to tone the entire hip, thigh and buttock areas, so you achieve a balance. These muscles are responsible for shape and firmness, and you should devote twenty minutes EVERY day to toning them.

— gluteals (buttocks)
— hamstring (back of thighs)
— quadriceps (front of thighs
— adductors (inner thighs)
— abductors (outer thighs)

Presentation

Making the most of yourself

Confidence needs a bit of help. You have a duty to make the best of yourself, and that means finding that stylish sense of who you are. People will always notice a woman who dresses well, walks well and has a ready smile. Having a slim, smooth bottom and legs is as much about making them appear slim and smooth as actually being slim. As any man will tell you, a women isn't more beautiful just because her thighs measure 56 centimetres instead of 70 centimetres. A woman who has style shines head and shoulders above the rest.

So the first thing to look at are the treatments you can give yourself. On the whole, they're not worth mentioning. There will always be a manufacturer who claims amazing results from their scientifically tested potion, and in those before and after pictures you can see a tiny difference in skin texture. But standing out in a cold wind will change your skin texture. Rubbing it with oil will change your skin texture. Sagging skin is part of the ageing process and you never saw an eighty-year-old with legs to die for. Creams, gels, lotions and pills don't work. Massage doesn't work particularly well, though I'm prepared to concede to salt scrubs as long as you do them yourself. Looking after the surface of your skin only does a fraction of what diet and exercise do, but they're worth a try. Your best hope while you are waiting for your diet and exercise efforts to show their benefits, is to achieve a lovely optical illusion, so we'll start with preparing for a beautiful golden, fake tan with a salt scrub.

The salt scrub

Do this in the evening, or whenever you have a chance to relax in loose clothing afterwards. It isn't a good idea to get dressed straight away as you will be oily!

There are many excellent scrub treatments on the market, but the best ones tend to be extremely expensive for what they are. At the time of writing, the two most effective cost £28 and £25 respectively and last for about 6–8 treatments, depending on how thorough you are. Being a long way from any shops and decidedly 'green' about using the car to go and buy more supplies, I read the ingredients and realized that they were little more than coarse salt and scented oils in a large jar which you can get your whole hand into. My version, using the better body oils from Decleor at £10 a time, still comes out at less that £13 for the same amount of salt scrub, but you can use any oil you fancy as long as it's reasonably greasy and you don't mind cleaning the bath or shower afterwards. The oil stays on your skin as a sheer film of scented softness and will leave it silky smooth and help in the war against cellulite! Here is my recipe.

— A packet of plain coarse sea salt, or a packet of Dead Sea salt which you can find in most health stores. Fill a large jar to an inch below the rim.
— Scented body oil – about a teacupful. Pour over the salt. It will all be absorbed. Alternatively, you can use almond, olive or coconut oil, or other favourite massage oils, available from outlets like the Body Shop.
— Give it a good shake, fasten the lid and keep inside your shower.

Here's how you use it:

Shower or soak yourself for at least five minutes with hot water. This softens your skin and helps your pores to open.

Using a sponge or ruffle mitt, soap yourself really well and have a good scrub. It is important to get yourself really clean before you start the salt scrub.

Switch off the shower. You don't want the salt to be washed off just yet. Take a good scoop of salt scrub and, starting on your left side, massage it into the lowest part of your buttocks, at the top of the thigh. With a hand on either side of your leg, scrub up and down briskly ten times. Count.

Move both hands to the side of your buttock and hip, then rub one hand across your stomach. Keep this movement flowing, you shouldn't have stopped. Scrub hard up and down ten times.

Moving your right hand back between your legs again, move the scrub down the back of your thigh. This time the movement is two circular movements, one hand above the other, right hand lower going anti-clockwise, left hand scrubbing clockwise. Count twenty fast movements.

Standing up straight, take another handful of salt in your left hand and stretch the left leg back a little. Using your left hand only, rub up and down with the flat of your palm the whole length of your buttock.

Take another handful of salt and repeat from the beginning. This is quite hard work and you should find yourself slightly breathless.

Repeat the whole thing on the right leg.

Finish by scrubbing lightly all over your body, to distribute the oils evenly.

Rinse off thoroughly. If you need to shave your legs, do so now while the oil can soften the blade's action. Rinse again.

Once out of the shower, pat yourself with a towel and dry the crevices between toes, legs and under the breasts, but do not rub yourself dry or you'll lose all those oils. The dampness will soon evaporate and leave your skin silky smooth.

Add more body oil or cream to really soften and moisturize your entire body. Rub this in thoroughly with firm movements.

The fake tan

The easiest way to make cellulite look better is to have a golden sheen to your skin. White legs look flabby however good they are. You might want to do the real thing, but unless you've got a tan already it's going to take too long to get one. Use a fake one all over to get you started and cheer you up when you look in the mirror.

I admit to being a complete expert at applying fake tan, having given up real sunbathing for the less ageing, bottled version about fifteen years ago. Apart from anything else, it's so much quicker! Do a new tan every 4–5 days. It sounds a complete bore, but believe me, it only takes around twenty minutes to scrub off the old tan and ten minutes to apply the new one, which is an hour a week. How brown could you get in one hour a week lying in your back garden?

Here's how to do it:

— Do it the day after your salt scrub shower. The scrubbing will leave slight abrasions on the surface of your skin – it's supposed to do that – but the tan will get ingrained in those abrasions and look terrible. That's why it's best to scrub in the evening so you can go to bed and not have to parade your white, 'naked' legs in front of everybody.

— Always start at your ankles. If you put the cream on your thighs first, it will get on your chest as you lean over to do your lower legs. Rest your leg on a chair. Put the same amount of cream on each hand, and work down the sides of your left leg first, in twin circular movements. Don't rub the cream specifically on your feet, but dash a little on top of the foot and rub it briskly, blending at the sides.

— Work up your leg, behind the thighs and round to the front, covering the knee and not forgetting the backs of your knees.

— Rub up as far as you can, including your extreme inner thighs and buttocks. Your bottom needs to be brown all over!

— Now take a small dry flannel or a small towel and quickly run it between your toes, rub lightly along your heels and Achilles tendon area and finally over your bent knee. The skin is so hard here that tanning creams settle into it easily and you'll be left with dark brown wrinkles that are a dead give-away! Finally, run both hands over your entire leg once more to blend. Repeat on the other leg.

— Using this guide, repeat for your whole body. Make sure you rub a dry towel under your arms and in the skin area of your armpits, as the tan can settle here too.

— Finally, wash your hands thoroughly, and I suggest using a generous handful of coarse salt or your salt scrub to really get rid of the tan which likes to settle in telltale places like the cuticles, under your nails and between your fingers.

End of Phase One

Phase One is over, and you've done brilliantly. If you've managed to get through it without a day's cheating, give yourself a pat on the back because it's really hard: the majority of people who start a diet on Monday give up by Thursday, so the thing to remember is that if you can get this far, you can do it again.

Take Phase One as a benchmark. Go back to it any time your weight loss stalls, your weight creeps up, or you're simply recovering from a holiday or an undisciplined period in your life. You'll soon restore order, lose those rogue pounds and stop cellulite that's thinking of settling with a brief return to Cellulite Busting!

Phase Two: Where do I go from here?

Coasting

You've done well and you're not going to backslide. You look good, you've got where you want to be, and though you'd rather go out for a good curry and envy the girls who look sensational on weekly blow-outs and all-night benders, you're not going to be one of them. You have more respect for your body than that, and a good time doesn't hang on how much food you managed to put away!

It's chic to have a little bit of a slimming regime going to maintain that great body. All the celebrities do it. They take it easy and have the Big Macs and KFCs when they've just got over a big project, but as soon as a film script lands on their doorstep they've got their running shoes on. Out comes the water and salad: it's time to get seriously beautiful again.

Phase Two is called coasting because it's effortless. Your foot is off the accelerator but you haven't applied the brakes. If you do need to apply the brakes, go straight back to Phase One for two weeks. This is your golden rule.

The big problem is not letting go of your diet to such an extent that you backslide completely. If there was ever a case for being psychologically robust, it's now. Having robust psychology means having a strong will. The big pitfall with a diet being 'over' is that you start getting slack and you let go of that tight hold on yourself. How many times have I heard the old cry, 'I just can't get back into it any more'?

Coasting still means being as disciplined as before, but I have helped you with the option of going back to Phase One for two weeks every time you let bad habits take over. It doesn't feel so bad – you're not on a long-term regime, just a couple of weeks – like going to a health farm. So what kind of diet is Phase Two?

More variety

This phase has more variety within the same food groups. For example, instead of not eating exotic fruits or saving them for your days off, you can now have them whenever you like. It's not a blank cheque to eat chocolate instead of having a fruit dessert because that's not a fair exchange.

More fun cooking

This is a great time to put your new regime into practice. If you used to live on takeaways or ready meals, you might not be into making your own meals, but this is where you can experiment. Puddings like my Banana and Tofu Dessert are incredibly easy to make, but a world away from those puffed up, chemical-ridden mousses you used to buy. In the new world of chic self-sufficiency, get baking bread – it's satisfying to do and streets ahead of the stuff you get in shops. Oh, and it costs pennies per loaf.

More calories

This might not be an attractive feature, but the calories were severely restricted on Phase One, down to 1,200 on some days and 1,500 on others. It depended which meals you chose. Your energy shouldn't have been flagging, but if it was you'll be able to make up for it on this phase. It's still up to you, but if you want a nice pudding or a cooked breakfast, you can have them. They only add around 300 calories to your day's total, keeping you well within the calorie recommendations for weight stability. So don't worry.

The exchange method

You're not going to eat more meals. That simply allows chaos to creep in again, and getting into the habit of eating those snacks and missing meals might be hard to break. You're going to exchange one of the rigid elements of Phase One for another similar food or meal. For example, in Phase One, I wanted you to eat potatoes with your evening meal. In Phase Two you can still have potatoes, or exchange them for something similar, like pasta.

This is the idea behind the exchange system and here are some other ideas:

In place of	Any day	1–2 times a week	Never
Standard breakfast	Special K	bacon and eggs	croissants
	Shredded Wheat	rice crispies	baguettes
	Weetabix	cornflakes	burgers
	Milkshakes		fried eggs
			fried mushrooms
			black pudding
			Frosties, Sugar Puffs and all other sugar-coated cereals

In place of	Any day	1–2 times a week	Never
Cellulite Buster Big Salad	multigrain sandwich with plain filling	cold pasta salads	cereal bars
	beans on toast	cold rice salads	crisps
		couscous	chocolate
		falafels	

In place of	Any day	Occasionally	Never
potatoes for dinner	pasta	thin pizza bases	pastry
	rice	fried potatoes	poppadums
	bread		fried bread
	noodles		dumplings

In place of	Any day	1–2 times a week	Never
fish or chicken	steak	bacon	corned beef
	lean chops	ham	salami
	game		fat on meat
	venison		battered fish or meat
	lean beefburgers		breadcrumbed fish or meat

In place of	Any day	1–2 times a week	Never
listed starters	add bread with soup or prawn dishes	garlic mushrooms	pâté

In place of	Any day	Occasionally	Never
puddings and desserts		crumbles	pies
		fruit cake	cheesecake
		oat flapjack	
		ice cream	

RECIPES

Some of these cellulite-busting dishes are not included in the 30-day menu suggestions in Phase One of your diet on pages 132 to 153, but they should give you an idea of what you can do with the permitted ingredients on your diet. For example, I have not used pasta in Phase One, but by the time you are into Phase Two you will be able to eat pasta and rice as and when you feel like a more substantial meal. Just remember to match your food intake to your energy expenditure: if you have a lazy day ahead, eat lightly. If you are packing for a cycling holiday – eat well!

People often say that they choose burgers and Chinese meals because they simply taste so much better and I can understand this. However, getting to grips with simple cooking methods should make a difference to how you view 'diet food' and I can promise you that nothing I make is ever elaborate. I do not love cooking but I do love nice meals, and all these recipes are my own creations.

Fish

Basic pan-frying

Put a knob of butter (about 7g) in a frying pan with a lid and add 1 tablespoon of hot water. Heat gently until the butter melts. Add the fillet of fish and close the lid tightly. Cook very slowly for 2–3 minutes on each side, turning once. The water will start to evaporate, leaving the butter. (Don't worry about the butter, because most of it will stay in the pan.) Turn up the heat a little. When slightly browned, test that the fish is cooked by cutting into the fillet – if should be a whitish pink for salmon and white, not opaque, for white fish, and feel flaky rather than rubbery as it does when raw. Put the fish straight onto a hot plate and serve with whatever accompaniments you have chosen.

Baked

This is basically the same idea as for pan-fried fish. It takes longer, but it means you can leave it and it won't spoil.

Put the fish into a foil tray with a lid or wrap it loosely in foil, and simply add a knob of butter (about 7g). Make sure to brush to top of the salmon with butter so it browns nicely. Add herbs like tarragon, thyme or basil, sticks of carrot, onions and courgettes/peppers/mushrooms. In other words, experiment to your heart's content!

Bake for about 20 minutes in a moderate to hot oven. For the last 10 minutes, remove the foil lid or open the parcel. Pile onto a plate and eat.

Poached

If you're really paranoid about using fat or if you are on a low-fat diet for medical reasons poach the fish instead, because you then don't need the butter. If you're cooking salmon put the fish in a foil tray or use foil as an envelope, add a tablespoon of water. Wrap or cover tightly and cook in a moderate oven for about 10–15 minutes. If you are cooking white fish use a cupful of skimmed milk instead of water and season lightly with black pepper and freshly chopped parsley. If you want a sauce, mix 1 tsp cornflour with a little milk and stir into a thin paste. Pour this into the cooking liquid when the fish is nearly cooked. It will thicken and you can then add more parsley and herbed sea salt.

Ideas for simple salmon meals

Salmon and Orange

Add the juice and zest of an orange to 1 or 2 fillets of salmon. Leave to infuse for an hour or so. Add a dot of butter and oven bake for 20 minutes.

Salmon and Spinach

Line an ovenproof dish with plenty of washed and well-drained spinach. Spinach cooks down a great deal so you will need a large bag. Dot with butter and season with sea salt and coarse black pepper. Lay a salmon fillet on top. Cover tightly with foil and bake in the oven for 20 minutes. The water from the spinach will steam the fish perfectly.

Creamy Salmon with Dill

Poach a salmon fillet in a large frying pan. When it is cooked put on a plate to keep warm while you add 1 tbsp half-fat crème fraiche to the juices remaining in the pan, bring to the boil and then add a handful of finely chopped dill. Pour over the salmon and serve with Cellulite Buster Small Salad (see page 63) or plain mashed potatoes.

Cold Salmon and Dill Mayonnaise

Make a dill mayonnaise by mixing half a portion half-fat crème fraiche (maybe 1 tbsp) with half a portion mayonnaise (see page 64 for portion sizes). Add a small handful of chopped fresh dill and parsley. Put a salmon fillet you cooked using the one-spare system on a plate and serve with 2 teaspoons of the mayonnaise on the side of the plate to dip your salmon into. This works well with lots of fresh sliced cucumber and 3 small boiled new potatoes.

Fresh salmon recipes

Pan-fried Salmon with Green Lentils

It is very easy to get tinned green lentils these days from the major supermarket chains, but if you can't find them, don't worry. Soak some dried lentils overnight and then simmer them until cooked (about 45 minutes to an hour), rinse and drain thoroughly, then keep in the fridge in a snap-shut container until you need them. Once cooked, they easily last a week.

7g approx. (a small knob) butter
1 fillet salmon
2 tbsp lentils
juice of half a lemon
sprigs of watercress
dill mayonnaise (see page 133)

Heat the butter very gently in a frying pan, add the salmon and cook very slowly, turning once. Test that the salmon is cooked thoroughly. Transfer to a hot serving dish and keep warm.

Add a little more butter to the pan, tip in the lentils and gently heat through. Fry the lentils stirring constantly as they only need warming through. Tip the hot lentils on to a plate and put the salmon on top and immediately squeeze lemon juice over it.

Garnish with sprigs of watercress and put a small blob of dill mayonnaise on top, or a blob of half-fat crème fraiche.

Salmon with Fruit and Nut Sauce

1 tbsp toasted almonds
14g butter
1 salmon fillet
zest and juice of ½ lime
medium-sized bunch white grapes, washed, halved and
    de-seeded
salt and black pepper
fresh coriander to garnish
lime wedges

Toast the almonds in a dry frying pan over a medium high heat, shaking the pan constantly, until they have turned a warm brown colour.

Heat the butter in a frying pan. Add the salmon and cook as for basic pan-fried salmon (page 133). Remove the fillets and keep warm.
Stir the zest and juice of the lime into the pan. Add the grapes and cook over a low heat for 2 minutes. Stir in the almonds. Season to taste.

Cook for a further minute. Pour the sauce over the salmon fillets, garnish and serve.

Suggested accompaniments: salad leaves, or a bed of peas.

Barbecued Salmon with Citrus

14g unsalted butter, softened
½ tbsp dill, chopped
½ clove garlic, crushed
salt and black pepper
1 orange, sliced, with skin on
1 large salmon fillet

Mix the butter, dill and garlic together and season. Dot small pieces of the herb butter onto one half of a large piece of baking foil and lay half the orange slices on top. Lay the salmon on top of them, cover with more orange slices and more pieces of butter. Fold the foil over the fish to make a loose parcel and seal the join well.

Make three angled slashes in the foil, top and bottom. Place on the barbecue and cook for 15–20 minutes each side.

Smoked salmon recipes

Smoked Salmon with Prawns and Grapes

50g seedless grapes
50g prawns
84g smoked salmon, cut in strips
1 tbsp fresh vinaigrette (see page 64)
juice and rind of half a lemon
1 tsp half-fat crème fraiche
salad leaves – any combination of watercress, lamb's lettuce, rocket or chicory
flat-leaf parsley, chopped

Halve the grapes and mix with the prawns and smoked salmon strips. Mix the vinaigrette with the lemon rind and juice, then stir in the crème fraiche. Toss the prawns, smoked salmon and grapes in the dressing and pile onto a bed of green salad leaves. Sprinkle with parsley and serve.

Smoked Salmon with Avocado and Pine Nuts

1 tbsp pine nuts, toasted
84g smoked salmon, cut in strips
½ avocado, peeled and sliced lengthways
salad leaves
vinaigrette made with walnut oil (see page 139)
flat-leaf parsley

Toast the pine nuts either by spreading them on a baking sheet and putting them into a very hot oven for five minutes and shaking the tray halfway through, or by putting them in a dry frying pan over a high heat with no oil and shaking them constantly to prevent burning.

Combine the salmon, nuts and avocado together. Toss the salad leaves in the vinaigrette and arrange on a plate and pile the other ingredients on top. Sprinkle with parsley.

Smoked Salmon with Pasta, Watercress and Dill

This is incredibly easy!

1 cupful dry pasta shapes
1 slice smoked salmon cut into strips
pinch of dried dill or (preferably) few fronds of fresh dill,
    chopped
1 large bunch watercress, stems removed
1 dsp half-fat crème fraiche
black pepper

Boil the pasta in plenty of salted water until cooked. Drain and return to the pan and put over a very low heat. Add the smoked salmon strips and stir thoroughly. The salmon will rapidly go pale. Then add the dill, watercress and crème fraiche and mix thoroughly. Season with black pepper. As the salmon is very salty, there is no need to add any salt.

Serve immediately on very hot plates.

Chicken

Basic pan-frying

Use 1 tablespoon oil. Brown the chicken on both sides over a medium-high heat, then turn the heat down and cook thoroughly. Test it is cooked by cutting through one piece – it should be white throughout with no hint of pink flesh.

Oven-baked

Brush one boneless and skinless chicken breast with oil, or marinate for a few hours in either oil and orange or lemon juice and zest, then oven-bake in a throw-away foil dish.

Ideas for simple chicken meals

Mediterranean Chicken

When the chicken is cooked, throw in half a tin of ready-chopped toma-toes and a handful of chopped red, orange and yellow peppers. The amounts do not matter much – just have as much or as little as you like. Season with oregano and garlic (if you like garlic) and serve either alone, or on a bed of 1 teacupful cooked rice.

Creamy Chicken

Pan-fry the chicken following the instructions above. When it is cooked, add 1 large dsp half-fat crème fraiche to the pan. Turn up heat and stir well. Throw in a handful of parsley, a little pepper and herbs.

Curried Chicken

Cut a chicken breast into strips and roll them in a mixture of ground cumin, garam masala and coriander, then fry gently in 1 tbsp oil until completely cooked. Squeeze the juice of a lemon over the chicken. Serve with rice and a mixed green salad.

Tarragon Chicken

Cook as for Creamy Chicken but also add a handful of fresh chopped tarragon leaves or 1 tsp dried tarragon to the pan and stir well. Spoon over the chicken.

Chicken with Vegetables

Stir-fry the chicken, remove from pan and keep hot. Quickly stir-fry some mixed vegetables such as mange-tout, carrot sticks, broccoli florets, bean sprouts, chopped red and green peppers or any other vegetables that take your fancy. The list is long and you may have as many as you like!

Just before serving, add a dash of soy sauce (it is up to you to decide how much you need). Put the chicken back in the pan and heat through.

Chicken Recipes

Grilled Chicken in Orange Marinade

Serves 1   Calories per serving: 210

150–200g skinless, boneless chicken breast
juice and rind of 1 large orange
1 tbsp olive oil
clove garlic, chopped (optional)

Place all the ingredients in an ovenproof dish, stir well to mix, cover with foil and refrigerate overnight if possible, for a whole day or a minimum of two hours.

Pre-heat the oven to 180°C/350°F/Gas 4.

Remove the chicken from the dish and place on a wire rack over a roasting tin in the oven. Cook for about 20 minutes.

Turn the grill to high, and finish off the chicken by grilling thoroughly on both sides until brown and slightly caramelized.

Alternatively pan-fry over a medium heat with the lid on tightly, turning once or twice to prevent it burning. This takes about 10 minutes.

Barbecued Chicken and Lentil Salad

½ cup (125ml) low-fat plain live yoghurt
1 tsp cracked black pepper

1 clove garlic, crushed
1 tbsp fresh basil leaves, chopped
½ tsp ground turmeric
1 skinless and boneless chicken breast fillet
cooking-oil spray
1 radicchio lettuce

For the lentil salad (this makes enough for 3–4 servings)
1 medium red pepper, chopped
1 medium yellow pepper, chopped
1 cup brown lentils (tinned are fine)

For the walnut oil dressing
½ tsp sugar
1 tsp mustard
⅓ cup balsamic vinegar
1 cup walnut oil

1 bunch lettuce leaves

Combine the yoghurt, pepper, garlic, basil, turmeric in a bowl, add the chicken and mix well. Cover and refrigerate for one hour.

Remove the chicken from marinade and discard the marinade. Heat a barbecue or a griddle pan and coat with cooking-oil spray, add the chicken and cook on both sides until browned and tender.

Meanwhile, mix the ingredients for the lentil salad together. Make the dressing by putting the sugar and mustard in a jug and stirring in the vinegar. Whisk in the oil until creamy. Mix 2 tbsp with the lentil salad.

Line a plate with torn lettuce leaves, slice the chicken thinly, put on top of the lettuce and top with the lentil salad.

Chicken and Asparagus and Chickpea Salad

Serves 2

1 tbsp pine nuts
1 tbsp sunflower oil
150g chicken breast cut into strips
dark green salad leaves, for example lamb's lettuce or watercress
2 dsp walnut oil dressing (see above)
1 dsp half-fat crème fraiche

8 asparagus spears
1 tbsp tinned chick peas

Put the pine nuts in a dry frying pan over a high heat and toast for a minute or so, shaking the pan all the time. Put aside.

Heat the oil in the pan and add the chicken strips. Cook slowly for about 5 minutes, turning a couple of times.

Meanwhile, line two dinner plates with salad leaves. Make a creamy vinaigrette by whisking the walnut oil dressing with the crème fraiche. Pour over the salad leaves.

When the chicken is cooked, transfer it to a warm plate and keep hot.

Put the asparagus spears and chick peas into the pan adding a little more oil if necessary. Put a lid on the pan and cook rapidly, shaking all the time. Put the chicken back in the pan. Toss thoroughly then pour onto the salad-leaf base.

Tarragon Chicken or Lemon Tarragon Chicken

Makes 2 portions

2 tbsp sunflower oil
½ onion, finely chopped (optional)
2 skinless and boneless chicken breasts, flattened
½ tsp dried tarragon or 1 sprig fresh tarragon, chopped
2 tbsp half-fat crème fraiche
coarse sea salt
black pepper
rind of 1 lemon, grated
fresh flat-leaf parsley, chopped

Heat the oil and, if using onions, fry them first, then add the chicken and cook thoroughly. Test that the chicken is cooked by cutting through the centre of one piece. It should be white with no hint of pink.

Add the chopped tarragon. Turn up heat and then add the crème fraiche. Season well. The chicken should now be coated in a caramel-coloured sauce. Add the lemon rind.

Turn out straight away onto a hot plate and garnish with parsley and serve with mashed potatoes, peas and sweetcorn or a salad.

Salads

Malibu Salad

For the dressing
1 large tbsp Greek yoghurt
1 tsp mustard
1 tsp brown sugar
1 tsp cumin powder
juice of 1 lemon
1 tbsp olive oil

1 skinless and boneless chicken breasts
¼ large cos lettuce, chopped
few whole sprigs of mint
1 tbsp large raisins
1 bunch mint, chopped

Combine all the dressing ingredients in a bowl and beat well.

Grill or charcoal-grill the chicken breast and put in the centre of a serving plate. Surround the chicken with lettuce and mint sprigs.

Spoon the dressing generously over the chicken and scatter with the raisins and chopped mint.

Peach and Chicken Salad

1 dsp pine nuts, toasted
1 ripe fresh peach, peeled, stoned and cut into 8 pieces
1 cooked cold chicken breast, cut into bite-sized pieces

For the dressing
1 tbsp half-fat crème fraiche
1 tbsp walnut oil
1 tbsp pesto
1 tsp lemon juice
salt and freshly ground black pepper

½ packet mixed salad leaves
fresh basil leaves

Put the pine nuts in a dry frying pan over a high heat and toast for a minute or so, shaking the pan all the time. Put aside.

Put the peaches and chicken in a large bowl.

Place the dressing ingredients in another bowl and whisk together until well blended. Pour the dressing over the peach slices and chicken and toss together.

Arrange the salad leaves in a shallow salad bowl and pile the peach and chicken mixture in the middle. Scatter the pine nuts on top. Garnish with basil leaves.

Salade Niçoise

This is simply a different way with tuna fish.

Makes 1 portion

> salad leaves as a base
> 2 tomatoes, sliced
> handful French beans, cooked and cooled
> small cold potato (about 100g) peeled, cooked and diced small
> ½ tin tuna fish in water, drained
> 1 hard boiled egg
> few pitted olives
> 1 dsp capers
> 1 tsp mayonnaise or 1 tsp vinaigrette (see page 64)

Line a plate with the salad leaves and tomato slices. Arrange the beans and potato over the base, then add the tuna. Arrange the hard boiled egg on the tuna, sprinkle over the olives and capers, and serve with 1 tsp mayonnaise or 1 tbsp olive oil dressing.

Busy day? – double up the potato portion.
Lazy day? – leave the potatoes out.

Vegetarian recipes

Basic Pan-fried Vegetables with Parmesan and Pine Nuts

> any amount of whatever crisp vegetables you like
> 1 tbsp vegetable oil
> 1 dsp half-fat crème fraiche
> 1dsp pine nuts, toasted
> 1tsp Parmesan, grated

Stir-fry the vegetables in 1 tbsp oil, until slightly seared and still crisp. When nearly done, add 1 dsp half-fat crème fraiche and turn up the heat. Toss the vegetables well.

Have a hot plate handy and turn the vegetables out onto it. Dry the pan with a piece of kitchen towel and sear the pine nuts quickly, then toss them over the vegetables, sprinkle with the Parmesan and eat immediately.

Variations
— After a lazy day / for a lazy day ahead: add a small salad of watercress, chicory and asparagus.
— After a hard day / for a hard day ahead: serve on a bed of mashed potato (using 42g potato per person and mashing only with milk and seasoning) or 1 cupful cooked pasta shapes, or 1 cupful cooked rice.

Baby Spinach, Potato and Egg Salad

This keeps well in the fridge, so it's fine to make the extra portions even if it is for one person.

    4 tiny new potatoes, washed and halved
    2 dsp olive oil
    1 tbsp white wine vinegar
    1 dsp half-fat crème fraiche
    1 hard boiled egg, quartered
    handful baby spinach leaves
    4 anchovy fillets, finely chopped
    1 tbsp Parmesan, coarsely grated

Combine the potatoes and 1 dessertspoonful of the oil in a large baking dish and bake, uncovered, in very hot oven for 25 minutes. Drain on kitchen paper and allow to cool.

Whisk the remaining olive oil with the wine vinegar and crème fraiche to make a creamy dressing.

Combine the potatoes, eggs, spinach leaves and anchovy fillets and toss in the dressing. Sprinkle with the Parmesan.

Serve with a mixed salad, or with peas and sweetcorn.

Grilled Vegetable Salad with Creamy Dressing

Makes 1 portion

2 medium (150g) potatoes
100g medium flat mushrooms
4 baby courgettes, sliced in half
handful carrots, cut into sticks
cooking-oil spray
1 tsp Cajun seasoning
bag of spinach
1 medium oak leaf lettuce

For the creamy dressing
¼ jar sun-dried tomatoes in their oil, chopped
1 tbsp half-fat crème fraiche
1 tsp fresh or dried oregano, chopped
1 clove garlic, crushed
1 tsp balsamic vinegar

Cut potatoes into 1cm slices. Boil, steam or microwave them until they are just tender, then pat dry with absorbent paper.

Coat the potatoes and all the other vegetables with cooking-oil spray and sprinkle with the seasoning. Cook the vegetables in a hot frying pan or roast them in a very hot oven until browned and tender.

Make the dressing by draining the dried tomatoes and chopping finely. Whisk the oil and vinegar together and then combining with all the other ingredients. The dressing is best made immediately before serving.

Drizzle the vegetables with the dressing and serve with torn spinach and lettuce leaves.

Vegetable Kebabs with Salsa

For the salsa (this will make one jar)
½ onion, chopped finely
½ red pepper, chopped finely
500g tomatoes, de-seeded and quartered
½ tsp allspice
½ tsp cayenne pepper

1 dsp vinegar
1 dsp soft brown sugar

For the kebabs
1 courgette, sliced thickly into 3cm rounds
few pieces red and orange pepper, cut thickly
½ onion, cut into thick pieces which will go on a skewer
1 carrot, cut into 3cm rounds
3–4 small cauliflower florets
3 small baby new potatoes, cooked but not peeled
3–4 baby corns
1 tbsp oil

Put all the salsa ingredients into a pan, except the vinegar and sugar. Cook on a low heat until soft, about 30 minutes. Then add the vinegar and sugar to the salsa and stir well. Simmer until pulpy, possibly a further 30–60 minutes depending on the ripeness of the vegetables you used.

Allow the salsa to cool, the spoon onto the plate. For best results with the salsa, make several jars, seal while still hot and keep for three months to allow the flavours to develop.

Thread the vegetables onto a skewer and brush with the oil. Grill the kebabs on a barbecue or standard grill, turning until soft but still crisp and golden.

Serve the kebabs with the salsa.

Fruit and Nut Slaw

Makes 6 portions (keeps well)

For the dressing
4 tbsp half-fat crème fraiche
4 tbsp olive oil
2 tbsp wine vinegar
2 tbsp water
2 tbsp lemon juice
1 tsp Dijon mustard
salt and ground black pepper

For the slaw
¼ medium red cabbage, washed, drained and finely shredded
¼ white cabbage, washed, drained and finely shredded

4 spring onions, thinly sliced (optional)
1 carrot, grated
2 red apples, peeled, cored and thinly sliced
20 brazil nuts, halved
10 walnuts, broken
8 tbsp raisins
handful fresh flat-leafed parsley, roughly chopped

Place all the dressing ingredients in a bowl and whisk well to combine.

Place the prepared vegetables, the fruit, nuts and raisins in a bowl and pour over the dressing and toss well.

Refrigerate for an hour to allow the flavours to develop. Serve garnished with chopped parsley.

Creamy Nut Salad

Makes 2 portions

The amount of vegetables you use does not really matter. Change the combination to suit your taste.

2 tbsp sunflower oil
medium potato, cooked and sliced into chunks
6 baby courgettes or 3 standard sized courgettes
1 large carrot, sliced or handful ready-made carrot batons
few broccoli florets
1 tbsp pine nuts
1 tbsp flaked almonds
1 tbsp creamy dressing (see page 64)
fresh coriander leaves
fresh flat-leafed parsley

Warm a plate.

Heat the oil in a large frying pan with a lid. Add the potatoes first, and cook for a minute, add the rest of the vegetables and turn down the heat. Put the lid on and shake well. After a minute, turn up the heat again to sear.

Tip all the vegetables onto the plate, wipe the pan dry and put it back on the heat. Add the pine nuts and almonds and toast well over a high heat, shaking the pan all the time.

Tip the nuts over the vegetables. Add the creamy dressing and sprinkle with parsley and coriander. Eat straight away.

Cottage Cheese and Fruit Salad

Makes 1 portion

    1 large tbsp or 1 small tub good cottage cheese (do not use the
        low-fat variety unless you have medical problems – a good
        creamy cheese such as Loseley organic is my favourite)
    ½ apple, sliced
    ½ banana sliced
    few kiwi slices
    ½ orange, segmented
    1 dsp blueberries
    6 grapes, sliced
    few chunks fresh pineapple
    ½ peach, sliced
    3–4 strawberries, sliced thinly
    1 whole orange (optional)

Put the cottage cheese in the centre of a dinner plate and arrange the sliced fruit round it. Alternatively, and for an impressive light lunch for friends, slice the top off an orange and scoop out the flesh. Spoon the cottage cheese into the middle of the orange. Slice the bottom so it will stand up without rolling over, and surround with the sliced fruit.

Waldorf Salad

    lettuce leaves or watercress
    1 stick celery, sliced
    ½ apple
    6 walnuts, halved
    6 grapes, halved
    1 dsp mayonnaise (see page 64)
    zest of an orange

Line a dinner or dessert plate with lettuce leaves or watercress.

Put all the other ingredients into a bowl except for the orange zest and toss well. Turn out onto the leaves and sprinkle the zest over.

Cellulite Buster Protein Shake

I defy anybody not to love this invention of mine. I don't agree with 'dashboard dining' – taking food with you to eat on the way to work – but if you have to, you won't go far wrong with this nutritious, delicious meal in a glass.

    1 tbsp porridge oats
    1½ teacupfuls skimmed or soya milk
    1 banana, sliced
    1 tbsp plain live yoghurt (I suggest Danone Activa)
    6 whole almonds or 6 walnut halves
    3 dried apricots, chopped
    1 tsp wheatgerm (Bemax or Froment)
    tiny pinch of cinnamon
    2 tsp honey

Put the oats and milk into a blender or food processor and leave for an hour or overnight (if you are having this for breakfast, I suggest you do it the night before).

Add the banana, yoghurt, nuts, apricots, wheatgerm, cinnamon and honey. Blend for a few seconds until completely smooth. Pour immediately into a glass and drink slowly. This will make more than one glass.

You can substitute a few chopped dates instead of the apricots and use walnuts. Figs and brazil nuts are another good combination.

Puddings and desserts

Peach, Blueberry and Cherry Fruit Salad with Kirsch

Makes 3–4 portions

    2 ripe peaches, washed, stoned and thickly sliced
    100g cherries, washed, stoned and halved
    175g blueberries, washed
    juice of 1 lemon
    6 tbsp kirsch
    25g flaked almonds, toasted
    crème fraiche to serve (optional)

Place the peaches, cherries and blueberries in a serving bowl.
    Stir the lemon juice and kirsch together and pour over the prepared

fruit. Mix gently, cover and chill thoroughly. Just before serving, sprinkle the toasted almonds over the fruit salad. Serve at once with crème fraiche, if desired.

Winter Fruit Salad

Makes 2–3 portions

    tin of prunes in apple juice
    12 dried apricots
    60g flaked almonds (optional)
    6 tinned figs
    1 banana, sliced

Put all the ingredients together in a large bowl, making sure the banana is covered by the juice. Store in the fridge and use for breakfast, as a dessert or as a topping for yoghurt.

Banana and Tofu Cream Dessert

Makes 4 portions – divide into individual bowls, cover and refrigerate until needed.

    1 large banana
    100g tofu (this is solid, and comes in either a block, or squares)
    50g ground almonds
    2 tbsp natural yoghurt
    2 tbs honey

Simply put all the ingredients into a blender, or use a hand blender (the mixture tends to be a little stiff) and blend thoroughly, divide into small pots and refrigerate.

Strawberry, Banana and Peach Kebab

If you haven't had much baked fruit, you're in for a treat. Barbecued fruit kebabs are a good place to start, and they're perfect for you and your children's diets.

Makes 2 portions

    2 bananas, sliced
    2 firm peaches, washed, stoned and quartered

12 whole firm strawberries
a little melted butter
1 tsp sugar for glazing
Greek yoghurt or half-fat crème fraiche or fromage frais, to serve

Thread the fruit onto wooden skewers and brush with the melted butter. (Most of the butter will drip off, don't worry.)

Place on a hot barbecue or under a pre-heated grill for ten minutes, turning frequently. Sprinkle with sugar as you turn the kebabs.

Place a pool of Greek yoghurt, half-fat crème fraiche or fromage frais on a side plate, gently ease the fruit from the skewers on top.

Baked Bananas

1 banana, sliced lengthways
juice of 2 oranges
1 tsp sugar
Greek yoghurt or half-fat crème fraiche or fromage frais

Put the banana into an ovenproof dish and pour the orange juice over. Cover with foil and bake in a hot oven for 10 minutes.

Take off the foil, sprinkle with sugar and put under a hot, pre-heated grill to caramelize.

Serve as for kebabs.

Baked Peach in Sherry

Makes 4 portions

4 ripe peaches, stoned and halved
4 tiny knobs of marzipan
1 teacup medium sherry
juice of 4 oranges per person
Greek yoghurt or half-fat crème fraiche or fromage frais

Slice the peaches and remove the stones. Sandwich the two halves together again with the marzipan – squeeze together tightly.

Stand upright in an ovenproof dish and pour the sherry and orange juice over. Cover tightly with foil and bake in a medium oven for 30–45 minutes. Test that the peach is soft throughout, the amount of cooking will depend on the condition of the peaches when you buy them.

Serve as before.

Tip the nuts over the vegetables. Add the creamy dressing and sprinkle with parsley and coriander. Eat straight away.

Cottage Cheese and Fruit Salad

Makes 1 portion

    1 large tbsp or 1 small tub good cottage cheese (do not use the
        low-fat variety unless you have medical problems – a good
        creamy cheese such as Loseley organic is my favourite)
    ½ apple, sliced
    ½ banana sliced
    few kiwi slices
    ½ orange, segmented
    1 dsp blueberries
    6 grapes, sliced
    few chunks fresh pineapple
    ½ peach, sliced
    3–4 strawberries, sliced thinly
    1 whole orange (optional)

Put the cottage cheese in the centre of a dinner plate and arrange the sliced fruit round it. Alternatively, and for an impressive light lunch for friends, slice the top off an orange and scoop out the flesh. Spoon the cottage cheese into the middle of the orange. Slice the bottom so it will stand up without rolling over, and surround with the sliced fruit.

Waldorf Salad

    lettuce leaves or watercress
    1 stick celery, sliced
    ½ apple
    6 walnuts, halved
    6 grapes, halved
    1 dsp mayonnaise (see page 64)
    zest of an orange

Line a dinner or dessert plate with lettuce leaves or watercress.
    Put all the other ingredients into a bowl except for the orange zest and toss well. Turn out onto the leaves and sprinkle the zest over.

Cellulite Buster Protein Shake

I defy anybody not to love this invention of mine. I don't agree with 'dashboard dining' – taking food with you to eat on the way to work – but if you have to, you won't go far wrong with this nutritious, delicious meal in a glass.

   1 tbsp porridge oats
   1½ teacupfuls skimmed or soya milk
   1 banana, sliced
   1 tbsp plain live yoghurt (I suggest Danone Activa)
   6 whole almonds or 6 walnut halves
   3 dried apricots, chopped
   1 tsp wheatgerm (Bemax or Froment)
   tiny pinch of cinnamon
   2 tsp honey

Put the oats and milk into a blender or food processor and leave for an hour or overnight (if you are having this for breakfast, I suggest you do it the night before).

Add the banana, yoghurt, nuts, apricots, wheatgerm, cinnamon and honey. Blend for a few seconds until completely smooth. Pour immediately into a glass and drink slowly. This will make more than one glass.

You can substitute a few chopped dates instead of the apricots and use walnuts. Figs and brazil nuts are another good combination.

Puddings and desserts

Peach, Blueberry and Cherry Fruit Salad with Kirsch

Makes 3–4 portions

   2 ripe peaches, washed, stoned and thickly sliced
   100g cherries, washed, stoned and halved
   175g blueberries, washed
   juice of 1 lemon
   6 tbsp kirsch
   25g flaked almonds, toasted
   crème fraiche to serve (optional)

Place the peaches, cherries and blueberries in a serving bowl.
   Stir the lemon juice and kirsch together and pour over the prepared

Bread

Before you dismiss bread making as something you only do when you haven't got a life, or have 2.4 children, you're behind the times. With more and more people living alone, there's never been a better time to master the art of baking just one loaf of bread. It's simple, it's unbelievably delicious, it's chemical free and it's your own. Try serving it up at a supper party to really impress your friends.

You can make one loaf of bread in a throw-away foil container so you don't even need a special tin. Unfortunately you can't make it without using a mixing bowl, but anything will do. And the real beauty of this and most of my other recipes is that you measure everything using a standard teacup, teaspoon, tablespoon and so on. Not a set of scales in sight.

I've given you three easy breads to try and a recipe for soda bread. You can also make your own recipes using almost anything. As long as you get the flour/yeast/salt/water combination right, you've got nothing to worry about. You can add olives, tomatoes, cheese, dried fruit – as long as you knead it for long enough. Kneading matters a lot.

Apricot and Brazil Nut Bread

I love this bread with a passion, especially toasted. You need to use a standard teacup for all measurements.

Makes one large loaf

    2 teacups plus 1 tbs strong plain white flour
    1 level tsp dried yeast (buy the activated yeast)
    1 level tsp salt
    2 tsp sugar
    ¼ tsp cinnamon
    1 teacup mixed broken brazil nuts and chopped apricots
    1 teacup warm water mixed with a little milk
    1 tbsp walnut oil or olive oil

Put all the dry ingredients into a large mixing bowl. It should be very large – if you're short of workspace, you can keep the dough in the bowl for the whole process of kneading. I use a cheap, round washing-up bowl which cost me £1.29.

Pour in the water/milk mix and the oil. Start to mix using your hand. If the mixture gets a little soggy, add more flour a little at a time. Gather the dough into a ball.

Knead for no less than ten minutes. This doesn't have to be a performance, but it has to be done. Kneading is done by pulling the outside of the dough towards the centre working your way round and round, so that you incorporate air. Flatten the ball, take the side furthest away from you and fold it in to the centre. Push the dough away from you to stretch it and turn it a quarter turn. Repeat. It might be boring but it's good exercise for your arms! When the time is up, leave the dough in the bowl, put a damp tea towel over the top and go away for an hour. If the room isn't very warm it might take 2 or 3 hours.

The dough should now be double the size it was. If it isn't, it has either been too cold or you put in too much salt. Nothing can be done about the latter, so throw it away and be more careful next time. Salt kills yeast!

Now you do what's called knocking back. It takes 30 seconds. You take the dough out of the bowl and press all the air out of it, pushing it back to the size it was before. Seems a waste, but the first rising stretches the gluten in the flour. Make it into a loaf-shaped sausage or a flat round, according to the shape of loaf you fancy. Put the dough on an oiled, floured foil tray or into a long foil loaf container. Cover it up and leave it to rise again for about an hour when it should be doubled in size again.

Pre-heat the oven to 400°F/220°C/Gas 7.

Put the bread straight in the oven to bake and about 20 minutes later, you should have one golden, fragrant loaf!

This all sounds laborious, but it isn't. Most of the work is the kneading, but most of the time is spent doing nothing at all. If you want to leave the dough and go out for the day, it will rise in the fridge, taking about 8 hours.

Multigrain Bread

This is made exactly as for Apricot and Brazil Nut Bread, but this time you use seeds instead of fruit and nuts. You'll need packets of pumpkin, sesame, poppy and sunflower seeds. In fact, buy quite a lot and keep them in the cupboard. This is one loaf you'll be dying to make again.

Instead of the apricots and brazil nuts, substitute a cupful of mixed seeds, varying the quantities according to your favourites. Leave out the sugar.

Plain White Bread

Make as above, but leave out the additions. You might need a little more flour.

Soda Bread

This is completely sensational, but you have to eat it straight away. You can freeze the dough and cook some later if you have a spare afternoon and want to make a batch.

> 2 cups strong white flour
> 1 pot (120g) plain live yoghurt plus 1–2 tbs milk
> 28g softened butter
> 1 tsp bicarbonate of soda
> 1 tsp cream of tartar
> ½ tsp salt

Pre-heat the oven to 230°C/450°F/Gas 8.

Grease a throw-away foil plate, or put some greaseproof paper on an oven tray to save washing-up. The foil plate should be the type you buy to make pies or quiches in – wide and deep-ish.

Mix everything together. It's as simple as that. Keep turning over with your fingers to make sure everything is incorporated. Cover your fingers with flour and shape the dough into a ball, flattening slightly.

Put on the tray or foil plate and cut a deep cross in the top. Put in the oven.

Keep checking, but it should be ready in about 25–30 minutes. Cool on a rack. I don't need to tell you to eat as soon as possible, because you won't be able to stop yourself!

Conclusion

It is important that you always put your body and its needs at number one in your life. It isn't obsessive. You're a delicate balance of energy and growth, health and fitness, and if any of these get out of whack the results can be devastating. You have rows with people you love, your work suffers and you feel embarrassed and stupid about doing the simplest things, like walking into a room or wearing a certain dress.

You can't have a healthy diet that only affects half of you. The food and exercise in this book will help banish cellulite but it will improve every bit of your body too. In eating well and rediscovering exercise, you're going to feel great. Your diet hugely affects your stress levels, and this diet is brilliant in its range of foods that directly affect mood. So you'll feel good and this will encourage you to get fit. Getting fit will make you look great and the whole happy cycle starts again.

My first big hit was my book *5 Days to a Flatter Stomach*. People still buy it and carry the book around with them so they have the diet at all times. I'm sure you're going to find this book just as useful. The section for your measurements will, I promise, become something you refer back to regularly, and the diet is easy to follow in the charts and tables.

Be proud of yourself. You have only one body and it's going to be with you longer than anyone else will. Keep up with this plan. You can look good for ever, and you will.

Good Luck!

You can write to Monica Grenfell at PO Box 58, Oxfordshire OX12 9BS
or visit her website at *www.monicagrenfell.co.uk* for more tips
and to purchase her other books and videos.